SACRED TEACHINGS
OF THE ASCENDED MASTERS

Daily Meditations,
Violet Flame Energy,
and
"I AM" Power Affirmations

SACRED TEACHINGS
OF THE ASCENDED MASTERS

****

A Compilation of Teachings
OF SPIRITUAL FREEDOM
from
Saint Germain and the Ascended
Masters

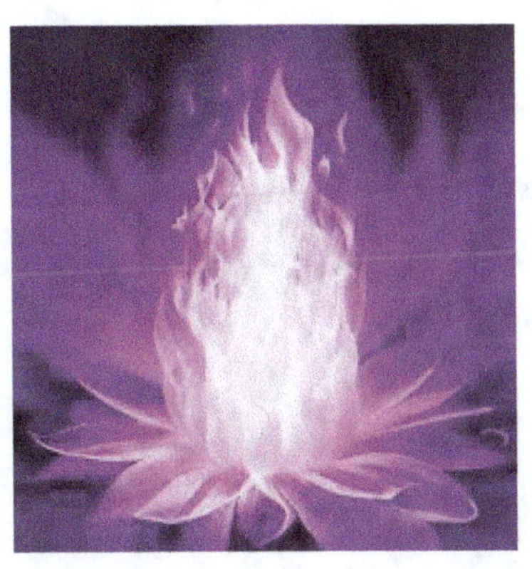

By
Marilena Mocanu

Marilena Mocanu

Today:

I have given this book to:

____

*Because I care about your well-being,
and I hope that these pages will inspire you for
achieving whatever you want.*

Signature:

Marilena Mocanu

*I would like to inform you that a part of
the revenues from the sale of this book will be
donated to schools in Romania, Spain, and the
United Kingdom helping to ensure that
children receive at least one nutritious meal
each day.*

*Thank you for your support, and I hope
you enjoy the book.*

With gratitude,

Marilena Mocanu

Dedication

To my beloved husband, Fernando,
whose unwavering love, support, and
encouragement make everything possible. You
are my rock, my inspiration, and the light that
guides me.
To my children, for their joy and endless love,
which fuel my heart and remind me daily of the
beauty of life.
To my dear friends, Jorge and Susana Aguire,
for your friendship, wisdom, and constant belief
in me. Your kindness and encouragement mean
the world.

This book is for all of you, who make this
journey worth walking.

CONTENTS

About This Book

This book serves as a spiritual manual that uses affirmations, daily meditations, and real-world applications of divine truths to help readers become closer to the teachings of the Ascended Masters. It gives guidance for spiritual and personal development as well as a methodical framework for interacting with the Seven Rays' heavenly forces, each of which is connected to a certain day of the week.

What You Will Discover:

Daily Meditations:
Sunday (First Ray): Blue and Crystal Flames of Faith, Strength, Power, Protection, and the Will of God.
Monday (Second Ray): Golden Flame of Wisdom, Illumination, Love, and Peace.
Tuesday (Third Ray): Pink Flame of God's Pure Divine Love and Adoration.
Wednesday (Fourth Ray): White Flame of Purity, Resurrection, and Ascension.

Thursday (Fifth Ray): Green Flame of Truth, Healing, Consecration, and Concentration.
Friday (Sixth Ray): Gold and Ruby Flames of Peace, Healing, Grace, and Ministration.
Saturday (Seventh Ray): Violet Fire of Mercy, Compassion, Invocation, Transmutation, and Freedom.

1.   The Violet Transmuting Flame:
A powerful spiritual tool for forgiveness, harmony, and transformation.
This section is divided into:
Part 1: The Holy Trinity, The Law of the Circle, The Law of Re-Embodiment, and an in-depth explanation of the Violet Flame.
Part 2: The Law of Forgiveness and the Law of Harmony, with insights into the Seven Bodies of Man.
Part 3: Group decrees and practical applications for spiritual growth.
Part 4: Guidance for directors of spiritual classes, including prayers and a benediction.
2.   Affirmations "I AM": Harness the power of "I AM" affirmations to align with divine truth, manifest positive outcomes, and unlock inner potential.

For those who are looking for balance, clarity, and a closer relationship with their divine destiny, this book is ideal. It empowers readers on their path to transformation by fusing timeless lessons, spiritual exercises, and useful tools.

This book, which offers insight and direction from the well-known Ascended Masters, is a lighthouse that may be utilised for individual meditation or in a communal context.

Introduction

Welcome to a life-changing adventure of spiritual development and awakening. In order to help you connect with the energy of the Seven Rays of Light, this book, Sacred Teachings of the Ascended Masters, provides a potent collection of meditations, affirmations, and divine wisdom. Connecting with these divine forces is possible every day, promoting spiritual awareness, empowerment, and personal healing.

The lessons provided here are intended to be actively experienced rather than only understood intellectually. Through the Seven Rays, each of which symbolises a distinct facet of divine light, the Ascended Masters, who are renowned for their deep spiritual understanding, impart their wisdom and affectionate energy. These energies provide you the means to realise your full potential, whether it is the violet flame of mercy and transmutation or the blue flame of faith and protection.

The Seven Rays are the subject of each chapter in this book, which also includes daily meditations, affirmations, and useful applications. These exercises are meant to promote inner calm, aid in healing, and deepen your relationship with God. The "I AM" affirmations are especially powerful instruments that enable you to improve your consciousness, make positive life choices, and assert your spiritual identity.

You will discover insightful teachings about the Seven Bodies of Man, the Law of Forgiveness, the Law of Harmony, and the Violet Transmuting Flame in addition to the daily routines. These lessons, which offer direction on how to lead a balanced and spiritually satisfied life, are age-old but incredibly applicable in the modern world.

Small enough to fit in your pocket or purse, this book is not just a spiritual aid but also a companion for your daily practice. It is made to be easily accessible wherever you go. These teachings can help you get a better knowledge of the divine energies that surround you and the purpose of your soul, regardless of your level of experience with spiritual practices.

I encourage you to welcome the insight of the Ascended Masters into your heart and let their lessons guide you. May the energies of the Seven Rays provide you with spiritual freedom, healing, and tranquilly, and may this book encourage you to live in accordance with your ultimate truth.

Preface

The Elohim, Archangels, and Chohans, representing one of the Seven Rays of Light that surround each person's Causal Body, are said to send their energies daily.

This booklet, which includes the motivational sayings of the Ascended Masters and suitable decrees for each day, was produced to assist students in their daily meditations. It is made to be tiny enough to fit easily in a handbag or chela's pocket, making it portable and useful anyplace.

This compilation aims to celebrate the Earth and all her evolutions while uniting the world's prayer force in support of God and His Divine Messengers. To ensure a balanced flow of energy, the fortunate Chohans employ the exact same language everywhere.

We decree that you will find joy and peace in participating in this worldwide meditation, knowing that other devoted souls are also engaged in this sacred service.

Who Was Saint Germain?

Known as the Ascended Master of the Seventh Ray, Saint Germain is one of the most adored and respected people in the spiritual world. His name is a byword for spiritual enlightenment, transformation, and freedom. Saint Germain, a divine teacher, and alchemist who is frequently referred to as the "Master of the Violet Flame," helps us overcome obstacles that stand in the way of our spiritual and personal development and leads us towards spiritual emancipation.

Saint Germain has offered his wisdom to individuals who are prepared to embrace greater consciousness throughout history, taking on several guises and names. He is thought to have had numerous lives, providing spiritual advice in a variety of capacities, most notably as Christopher Columbus, Merlin, and Rama. Saint Germain has taught lessons of immense importance through these previous incarnations, assisting humanity in progressing towards higher planes of existence.

The Benefits of Learning from Saint Germain

When we connect with the teachings of Saint Germain, we are gifted with invaluable tools for personal transformation. His wisdom helps us unlock the power within to:

Transmute negative energy: Saint Germain releases us from fear, uncertainty, and limitation by teaching us how to change negative feelings, ideas, and experiences into positive energy through the Violet Flame.

Achieve spiritual freedom: He demonstrates how to release ourselves from the bonds of self-imposed constraints so that we might realise our full potential and lead happy, purposeful lives.

Align with divine will: We can discover our genuine path, fulfil our spiritual goal, and connect our lives with the divine purpose by studying his teachings.

Manifest abundance and healing: The manifestation of plenty, both spiritually and materially, is another fundamental component of Saint Germain's teachings, which enables us to live in accordance with the laws of the universe.

Why Learn from Saint Germain?

The wisdom of Saint Germain is timeless and useful. His teachings are intended for everyone who aspires to a closer relationship with God and themselves, not only those who are already spiritually mature. We can break free from outdated thought patterns, mend emotional scars, and build a solid spiritual foundation by studying Saint Germain. His teachings are a priceless tool for anyone pursuing self-realization and spiritual liberation because of his capacity to enable people to take control of their spiritual development.

You will discover the life-changing potential of Saint Germain's teachings and their significant impact through this book. It is a call to embrace who you really are, transcend your limitations, and pursue enlightenment and spiritual liberation.

SACRED

DAILY MEDITATIONS

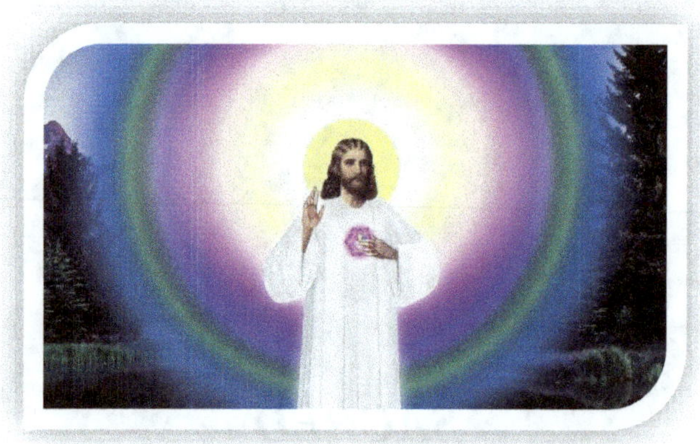

1.

---

§UNDAY
FIRST RAY BLUE AND CRYSTAL
FLAMES
OF
§TRENGTH POWER
PROTECTION WILL 0F GOD

---

1. EL MORYA, CHOHAN OF THE FIRST RAY OF GOD'S WILL: Beloved, it is the Heart of God I represent! The holy concept that I constantly transmit using the force of my attention arises from it. All I must do is tune into God's heart, and the flow begins and never stops! Focus on God's perfection while you relax in the diamond heart of your own perfection. The Will of God is divine order in all things; divine love expressed through all life; divine unity with the eternal source of all life - the One God - from whence we came. BE STILL and KNOW that **I AM GOD! I AM** that **I AM,** and **I AM** is all there is!

2. BELOVED PRESENCE OF GOD - "I AM" WITHIN MY HEART, I love and adore I summon You forth to blaze the Crystal and Blue Flames through me and see that God's Will is made manifest in all I do this day. I now realize that within my own heartbeat is God's Divine Plan for me and the way and means of bringing it into outer manifestation. I now enter the SILENCE and Listen; and I know the perfect thing to do. As I hold my attention upon the Divine Plan. I bring it into form.

3. "I AM" the **FAITH** in the **ALL-POWER OF GOD IN ME TO DIRECT** me, protect me, illumine me, heal me, supply me, sustain me, and do whatever **I REQUIRE TO HAVE DONE**

4. THE MORE YOU THINK OF, AND DO, GOD'S WILL ... the more your Threefold Flame will expand, and the centre of your being will join with the centre of all life. Your heart is the foundation of awakening, which originates in the spirit world. Let go and move forward with greater faith!

It is the Kingdom of Heaven within you, therefore as I shine a ray of light into your heart flames, take it in and absorb it, feeding the holy flame. Project this light—our united light, love, and power—out into all life on this planet and spread it throughout your four lower vehicles on the outbreath. Feel the Earth as a blazing diamond heart of God's Perfection, and accept it done right now and eternally sustained!

5. THE RELEASE OF GOD'S GIFTS, powers, and miraculous working presence into your world and affairs will begin with the simple recognition and realisation that God's presence is within you, waiting for an invitation to intensify it, according to **BELOVED LADY MIRIAM**, who is currently the Chohan of the First Ray. Your heart is alive with this **Ever-Presence**. To call it forth, you do not need a mediator. The solutions to our everyday issues are revealed by the comfort, calm, understanding, and directed intellect that emanate from its beautiful Self.

6. BELOVED LADY MIRIAM, for everything you have done for me and for all of humanity, I love, bless, and thank you. Now, envelop me in the blue flame of your love and give me your strength and ability to receive God's ideas and make them happen for the benefit of my fellow humans. let me to sense and comprehend Your Illumined obedience to that Will and the Presence of God within every human heart! I ask my beloved God Presence to let me say, *"Not my will but Thine be done I."*

7. THE GREAT ARCHANGEL MICHAEL - The Archangel of Protection and Defender of the Faith, asks: **"Through the Light of My Heart and your heart,** do We create for you through this appearance world NOW a Pathway of Love, Peace, Comfort, Opulence, Illumination and Well-being - physical, emotional, mental, and spiritual, Will you **FEEL** the Light of your heart creating this Path before you as you leave your room every morning and **WALK IN THE WAY OF THE**

ANGELS through the day in the exact same security as though you passed through one of the Rays which have been made an eternal pathway through the substance of the **Earth by the Masters**?"

8. ARCHANGEL MICHAEL, Protector Er Defender of the Faith: Beloved ones, you are a being of great light! I will fill you with my trust in the everlasting victory of God's First Cause of Perfection for all life if you allow me to enter your hearts. For a clear understanding of your own declaration of being, enter the Silence and make an appeal to your Presence. Discover your unique God Quality and mission, then try to live it out every day, in every circumstance. When you truly begin to live your part of the Great Divine Plan, all endeavours shall express the joy and enthusiasm of the Octaves of Light.

9. BELOVED ARCHANGEL MICHAEL, Send Your Ascended Angels of Protection to envelop me, my loved ones, and all good people on Earth, and to free us from thoughts and emotions that are not **God's perfect** concept for us. I love, bless, and thank you for **Your mighty** service to me, all humanity, and our planet for so long.

10. THE GREAT ELOHIM HERCULES says: "Are you happy with who you are and what you have manifested today?" Would you rather eat a whole loaf than only half of one? Are you happy to live in bodies of decay and limitations? You will create what you **WILL!** The Flame of Hercules burns on your forehead, dear students of Light.

Before you engage in the activities of the outside world, remember it every morning, acknowledge it, and **WILL** become what God has intended.

Remembering Hercules as you move forward, please do not accept such limitations in your individual selves when you know that **IT ONLY REQUIRES** the exercise of the **WILL WITHIN YOO** to draw forth **ALL THAT YOU REQUIRE!"**

11. THE PERFECTION OF GOD'S GLORIOUS KINGDOM OF LIGHT is all around you especially within the heart of the sacred fire. Make the thing that lives at the core of your existence consciously visible in the world around you. To achieve all your goals for your life and the world, put your faith in **God's First Cause's** perfection. Invoke my faith through your own chalice of consciousness into the **I AM** Presence of every life stream whose aura touches your own. In the

Name of the Light of God know that as you act to increase the faith of another, my own joy in service shall be yours!

12. BELOVED HERCULES I appreciate your tremendous service to our planet and everything on it, and I will continue to adore and bless you. Always give me unwavering protection by energising my physical, etheric, mental, and emotional bodies with the power of your love and the strength of my armies.

13. HERCULES, ELOHIM OF STRENGTH: The **ONE** Supreme Source of All Life, the **I AM** Presence, is the strength and power of the First Ray. Only the highest perfection is ever held and recognised by the **Father-Mother God**, who with great wisdom allows the very substance of their being to flow to all life everywhere. Each time you call on us, your awareness increases. The more time you devote to your spiritual nature, calling to your **I AM Presence,** the more rapid will be your development. With each such call you make, you **"open, expand, and strengthen"** your channel to the **Octaves of Light!**

14. IN THE NAME OF THE PRESENCE OF GOD WHICH "I AM", in the Name of Hercules,

WILL TO BE GOD-FREE in my mind, feelings, body, finances, world and affairs. **WILL TO BE GOD-MASTER! I WILL TO BE GOD INCARNATE!**

15. Continue to open your consciousness to our loving assistance, and as you do this more consistently, become more aware of yourselves as the children of God that you truly are. Learn how to integrate your divinity so that you can consciously participate in God's abundant creative manifestation!

Because the only strength and power I possess is **I AM.**

You possess spiritual strength, which allows you to completely control your body, mind, and soul in all actions. I counsel you that on awakening, daily and reverently turn your attention to the Presence of God within. As you do this, you will become a natural activity of service, for you have been called to be a **Presence of The Mother-Father God.**

16. PRINCIPAL, LORD OF DIVINE ORDER: I AM Divine Principle. I have clothed myself in a cloak of individualized consciousness and come forth from the Great Silence. **I AM** the **Flame of**

the **Great Central Sun,** and of the **Sun beyond the Sun.** I speak to you from the **Great Silence.** As I enfold you, I ask you to enter the Silence. You can locate me there and become one with everything I am! Then you will truly discover the divine essence from which you originated and from which **I AM.** You will feel a limitless feeling of delight if you can let go and ask God to take charge. A human being is the manifestation of Spirit in the material world. Your main goal is to develop the ability to summon the Spirit is gifts and make them material. Begin to believe in your own light, and to command that light! Begin each day with the command, **"I AM that I AM!"** Thus, do you place yourself in the flow of God's Light.

17. BELOVED PRESENCE OF GOD I AM within my heart; I love and adore you! I summon you forth to blaze your crystal and blue flames through me and see that **God's Will** is made manifest in all I do this day. I love, bless, and thank all the beings of light from the First Ray, who assist me this day. As God's most holy name ... I AM.

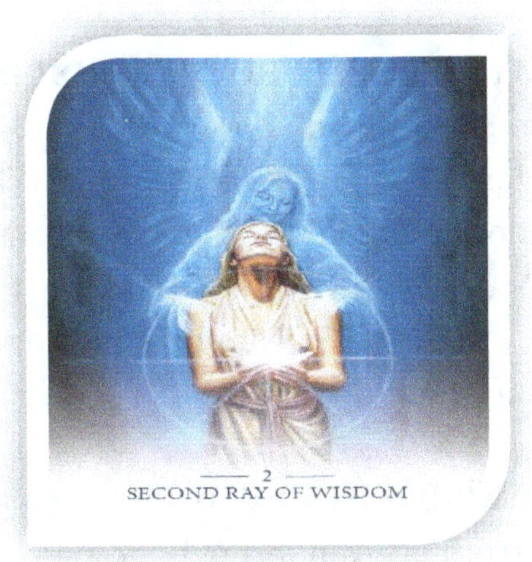

2.

MONDAY
SECOND RAY GOLDEN FLAME
OF
WISDOM ILLUMINATION LOVE
PEACE

---

l. MY BELOVED HOLY CHRIST SELF - "I AM" in me, I love and adore You! I summon forth the Golden Flame of Cosmic Christ Love and Illumination to enfold me this day. **"I AM" GOD'S ILLUMINATION AND WISDOM** directing me in all I do. I listen, and I understand, and I bless everything I contact this day.

2. DWJAL KHUL, CHOHAN OF SECOND RAY: All truth is given through the **I AM Presence** and released from the **Holy Christ Self** within your heart centre when your consciousness is open to receive. You see the evidence as a chela that humanity is realising the divine inside themselves. Understand that these information and truth come from the depths of your own actual self and reality. Please listen to me sincerely. Never forget that every day presents a fresh chance. Ask your Beloved God Presence, what is the next step? What would you have me do? Ask to see the divine principle involved and when this is clear in your mind and heart, move forward fearlessly.

3. I now understand that the **HEALING FLAME** that rids me of all my flaws is ALIVE within my physical body. I now understand that the **INFINITE SUPPLYING POWER** of all my needs and requirements is ALIVE within my physical body. I now understand that the **ILLUMINATION** of my outer consciousness is alive within my physical body, and that the **INTELLGENCE** that makes all form give to me the perfection that is within its own fundamental nature is **ALIVE** within my physical body.

Now I know that God is the only power in my heart, and that power acts for me in accordance with my faith in it. Thus, **"I AM"** in me, my **Holy Christ Self, COME FORTH** and allow your Divine Plan to happen.

4. BELOVED LADY SOO CHEE, now, according to Chohan of the Second Ray, each unique life stream arrived on Earth with a lovely lotus, which he was tasked with nurturing and bringing to full bloom into a spectacular blossom. He takes a petal from a flower and says, **"HE LOVES ME, HE LOVES ME NOT,"** as you have heard children do repeatedly.

5. At the end of each embodiment, there was only a bare stem with one or two petals in the core, which is what has transpired over the millennia by life streams. They then seen what had been done to their Beings' flower on the

"Other Side" and made a solemn pledge to return and tend to the Lotus. Please picture yourself now. Simply remove your human awareness and enter the vast Lotus of Our Retreat. Then, you will see the great **Master Beloved Confucius** softly guiding you into the extremely precious Petals of the Golden Lotus of Wisdom.

6. Allow the Holy Essence to just enter your mind; do not ponder about your inferior vehicles; instead, allow the elixir to flow organically through your mind; may the Golden Light fill your entire being, later you will say **"THANK YOU GOD, I LISTENED!"**

7. BELOVED LADY SOO CHEE, I appreciate your wonderful service to me and all of humanity, and I love and bless you. To bless and uplift all of humanity, may the Great Flame of Wisdom and Illumination from Your Golden Lotus Retreat spread through the Lotus of our Beings.

8. The most important thing is to do your absolute best! What your absolute best is truly known only to your Holy Christ Self and the ascended one with whom you are working. I pray that you consult the Master who resides in your heart for guidance while you work with the Octaves of Light.

9. BELOVED ASCENDED MASTER LANTO *"In your newfound service, you frequently feel the ingratitude and indifference of mankind, and sometimes you weary of well-doing,"* says **"World Teacher,"** the patriarch of the Rocky Mountain Retreat. We often feel discouraged when we stand in your surroundings. Then, would you kindly keep in mind those of us who have served you for millions of years, loving you, blessing you, and placing our trust and faith in you? Knowing this, you will take pleasure in restoring equilibrium to life by maintaining the same level of faith, patience, and confidence in your fellow humans."

10. BELOVED LANTO, you have served our planet for so long, and for that I love, bless, and thank You. Give us all the love that helps release it and the enormous **REVERENCE YOU HAVE FOR EVERY LIFE.**

11. BELOVED JOPHIEL, The Archangel of Illumination states: "I teach the consciousness to find the **POWER OF LIGHT WITHIN ITSELF.** That is my service to life. In the Second Sphere, concepts solidify and acquire shape. An abstract concept is given to you for your mind would think, **"I would like a home of eight rooms with an acre of ground,"** as Lanto is now the new home of World Teacher. Your emotions flow into the shape if the idea appeals to you, and the pressure of your emotions gives it vitality and manifests it.

12. JOPHIEL, ARCHANGEL OF ILLUMINATION: Beloved children of light, your I AM Presence is a seed, which strings forth when the soil is fertile, and the environment is pure. The fire of compassion and empathy is one of the most crucial instruments for preparing the soil in the garden of your heart. After your lotus has flowered, it is also used to keep it flawless and pure. As this takes place, your Holy Christ Self bursts forth, pouring forth its sweet essence into the grail of your consciousness. Then you realize the unmeasured service to life your divine soul has given.

13. BELOVED JOPHIEL, I appreciate your devotion to me and to all of humanity, and I love and bless you. Give me your sense of God's power within my own heart so that I may master every situation I encounter with the help of external light and love. You should also teach me how to externalise the divine ideas from God's heart into the outside world.

14. I bring to you my full momentum of illumination, wisdom and understanding. I invite you to breathe deeply, acknowledging and embracing the holy breath as the transformative force that will lead to enlightenment! Experience the first breath of life as the Holy Spirit is presence envelops you. Light is brought about by the love that pours out of your human heart. Feel 1t quickening the sacred temple of your body, as you release the breath. Accept the clarity of consciousness activating your mind and feelings.

15. BELOVED CASSIOPEIA, Perception and active, illumined contemplation of God's plan and design are the goals of the Second Ray, according to Elohim of Wisdom. Once you have decided to DO God's will, you must then receive the Divine Ideas, which are the instructions on HOW to make it happen. Being still is, therefore, the first thing the mind does after deciding to do something! The Golden Flame of Illumination, which will reveal Truth to you, lies within your heart.

16. Each morning as you awaken, say to your Presence: *"Mighty I AM Presence, take* *command of this outer self this day! Take command of every thought, feeling, spoken word, action, and reaction!"* Know that you are calling the wisdom of your inner Christ Consciousness while you do this, and that God's Divine Ideas will inspire you throughout your days! This is the reason for your being ... to become a conscious co-creator, to draw life's energy, to shape it according to your own God Design, to take these designs which are the ideas of the Father-Mother God, to plant them within your consciousness and bring them to fruition.

L7. BELOVED CASSIOPEIA I love, bless, and thank You for all You mean to our Earth and all humanity. Help me to follow through ' this Science of Precipitation and manifest each day some consciously externalized idea which I have thank You received from the Heart of the Father.

18. CASSIOPEIA, Elohim of Wisdom: My Temple is within the aura of the **Great Central Sun,** but it is also firmly anchored in the centre of your brain, by a bridge of light lovingly built by you. You embark on a journey of enlightenment, the road to your own mastery, as you collaborate closely with the **Ascended Masters** and the entire Spiritual Hierarchy. It is a turning moment in life, a shift in awareness, a growing awareness of the needs of all living things.

The external manifestation then turns into accepting responsibility for your own life energy use. You have within yourselves the will to do! I now offer you divine perception, so you may more perfectly fulfil your part in **God's Great Divine Plan**. The responsibility of expanding and projecting forth my gift to Earth now also becomes yours. You have advanced to a point where work such as this is possible for you to fulfil.

19. LORD LANTO, Patriarch of the Rocky Mountain Retreat: True reverence for life has within itself only the recognition of the purity, sanctity and perfection of the life force accorded to each one and that life force is God! Always remember that the breath is holy as you come to understand your oneness with all life. Of all the elements, the breath is the most sacred. Every breath you take qualifies it with your own ideas and emotions before it is exhaled and absorbed by all people. Let their abide within your heart the ever-present silent mantra: *God loves me, and I love God.* Hold this mantra within your mind. Where your attention is, there you are, for you are your consciousness. Where your attention is, your energy flows and your energy are your life. **GOD LOVES ME AND I LOVE GOD, AND I AM ONE WITH GOD!**

20. BELOVED PRESENCE OF GOD I AM IN ME; I love and adore you! On this day, I call forth the golden blaze of illumination to surround me. In a moment, I listen and comprehend, and I am guided by God's illumination and wisdom. All the beings of light from the Second Ray who help me today have my love, gratitude, and blessing. As God's most holy name ... **I AM.**

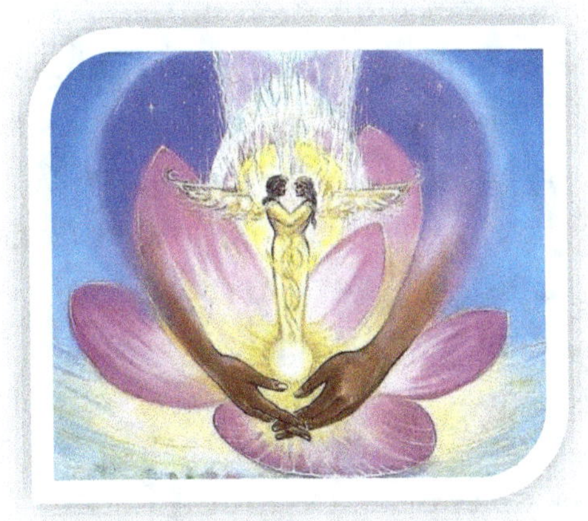

3.

TUESDAY
THIRD RAY FLAME PINK
OF
GOD'S PURE DIVINE LOVE
AND ADORATION

---

1.   **BELOVED PRESENCE OF GOD - "I AM" IN ME,** I love and adore YOU! I continuously offer my love and adoration to You, the Great God of the Universe, and His Messengers, oh, great and powerful flame within my own heart. I send my love to every living thing on the planet. With every thought, emotion, phrase, and deed I encounter today, I bless all life. On this day, I do not condemn, judge, or criticise! By word or deed, I FORBEAR to live my life without the full blessing of God.

"I AM" SEALED IN GOD'S PINK FLAME OF LOVEI "I AM" THE COMFORTING PRESENCE TO ALL LIFE EVERYWHERE!

2.   **BELOVED PAUL, THE VENETIAN,** "Come with me today away from the worries of the outer self, enter with me into that chamber **WITHIN YOUR OWN HEART, THE SECRET PLACE OF THE MOST HIGH,"** says the Maha Chohan, a former Chohan of the Third Ray. *"While you stand there, contemplate the Three-fold Flame, which is the garment of your own beautiful Christ Self, just relax in the Love of the Presence of God."* As your devotion flows to that Presence, keep in mind that your body is the Temple that contains the Immortal Flame of Eternal Life and the Christ Self, created in the image and likeness of the

Eternal, waiting for your dedication, love, and admiration. To the extremely few who do seek its help.

It says: My Beloved **ALL THIS YOU ASK I CAN BE - ALL THIS AND** More I Beloved ones, when your adoration becomes the **CONSTANT** activity of your innermost self, this Christ Self will grow - will expand. You will not have to say anything to declare it. As your life is poured into it, the **LIGHT** that is growing from the ever-increasing Presence will respond, creating a brilliant and radiant aura about you that **EVERYONE WHO RUN MAY READ IT.**

3. BELOVED PAUL, THE VENETIAN, I love, bless, and thank You for all You have done for me and for all humankind. Teach me to be the GENTLE-man (the GENTLE-woman) and to be endowed with your Gifts of Tolerance, Tact, Diplomacy, Forbearance, and the **ABILITY TO GET ALONG WITH MY FELLOWMAN!**

4. LADY ROWENA, CHOHAN OF THE THIRD RAY: The way of love is a path of service and silence. Embrace the silence ... of looking within with com passion and love toward yourselves and everyone you meet upon your path. We are going to guide you as you go along, and it is your duty to understand and accept that we are constantly by your side.

Now, in silence, close your eyes and let your mind to rest in the secret and priceless garden of your heart. The pink rose of love is securely blossoming inside your heart, and I am here. Nurture this rose carefully and constantly, until its aura of beauty and love expands, completely always enfolding you.

5. BELOVED LADY MASTER ROWENA, The Third Ray Chohan states: *"To become centred within the immortal Victorious Three-fold Flame within your heart assures the individual **FREEDOM** from all that is less than Christ Perfection,"* Because the more a somebody practices an action, the more proficient they become, it is crucial that the chelas under our supervision do this exercise every day.

It is, or should be, the goal of everyone under the per- sonal supervision of the Ascended Masters of Wisdom and Cosmic Beings to attain the Spiritual Status of the Christ in action at all times - allowing that glorious Being to be the Directing Intelligence in all your actions. *"It is of the utmost importance that the chelas avail themselves of the radiation and blessings of the*

Third Ray by contemplation of Its activity of Pure Divine Love and the Balance contained within it."

Being the Christ in action in the world of form means working with your spiritual advisors to provide wise counsel while adhering to the guidelines of the **Holy Christ Self** to bring Illumination in your own beings and worlds, and to be radiating centres of **PURE DIVINE LOVE** for the evolutions of this Earth, *"Oh, dear friends, I assure you that once you have truly experienced the Christ Way of Living, all else fades into insignificance and you become ONE with US who are ONE with Life in all its manifestations - remembering always that to attune one's self with the ONENESS of all is to become identified with the Perfection which exists in all manifestation, for all existence contains within it the active Principle of the Father-Mother God!"*

6. DIVINE LOVE EMBODIED IN YOU, beloved ones, is a full atonement with the celestial love at all levels of consciousness and through this ever-expanding stream of light you will find the pathway of understanding the virtues and qualities of pure divine love, for divine love embodies the first principle of creation ... that all life is one! Understanding the numerous difficulties and trials you face on your journey to self-mastery is tempered by divine love. Dear ones, bring the divine will of our **Father-Mother God** to life with ease and gentleness by using subtlety and tenderness in the expression of heavenly diplomacy. You will then receive the gifts of joy and happiness in return for expressing this way of being!

7. BELOVED LADY MASTER ROWENA, for everything you mean to me and to all of humanity worldwide, I love, bless, and thank you. Assist me in maintaining my focus on the **Holy Christ Self**, which is rooted in my heart, so that I can fully perceive its immense perfection in all that I do, think, say, or feel in my worldly and personal concerns.

8. BELOVED ARCHANGEL CHAMUEL Archangel of Adoration says: *"The Adoration Flame is practical! It is one of the most practical activities that can be generated within the heart; soul and spirit of the bound because it is an actual treatment of the feelings as well as of the mind, and an actual **THERAPY TO THE FLESH!** True Adoration to God has within it no self-seeking It is complete rest, enjoying God's goodness and adoring Him for who He is, or loving any great God-being who symbolises a unique contribution to life."*

I challenge any individual in de- pression, any individual in pain, any individual in chains of any kind to use the **FLAME OF ADORATION** that is the true nature, of their being. If, in using that, they do not see and feel **FREEDOM**, then the Sun and the planets themselves will no longer move on their appointed courses,"

9. BELOVED CHAMUEL, For Your wonderful help to me and to all of humanity, I adore, bless, and thank You. Fill my world and myself with Perfection by igniting Your Pink Flame of Adoration in every cell of my body. Blaze Your **PINK FLAME OF ADORATION** through my finances and my supply of money, and cause it to expand into my financial freedom, Blaze Your **PINK FLAME OF ADORATION** through my feelings that they may expand the **LOVE OF GOD** until it becomes all the life I contact. in a Pillar of the Pink Adoration, Comfort, and a contagion to Keep me sealed Flame of Love, Perfection.

10. HOLY AEOLUS, Cosmic Holy Spirit: I AM the protective, loving power of Holy Spirit, descending always from your beautiful **Presence of God I AM!** I descend in tongues of living flame! I fill your entire being with the flame of my Presence, of my peace and my love. Love is the unifying element, the basis that each individual needs—yes, needs—to return to the Heart of the **Great Universal God,** the creator of all life. There is only the ONE Path in that sense and comprehension.

To fan the creative fire inside your heart into a powerful blaze that will unite all life on Earth with the love of the Cosmic Holy Spirit, I breathe my flame of perfect love and tolerance into it! Now, expand my glowing pink flame from the centre of your heart as you breathe it in.

Become **ONE** with every life stream! You are **ONE** in love, **ONE** in desire, **ONE** in service, **ONE** in loyalty ... Loyalty only to the **PRESENCE OF GOD I AM** within your heart. Take time to enter the Silence and receive the gentle Love of God and within this Wisdom realize that *"balance is the key!".* Allow me to fill your souls with my unconditional affection.

Think about the Holy Spirit is grace and silent blessings that permeate everything so continuously. In all your living, emulate the pure and silent white dove which is the expression of the activity of the Holy Spirit.

11. THE GREAT ELOHIM - ORION - says: "I bring to you, individually, the fullness Of the PINK FLAME AND RAY". I offer it as a spiritual alchemy that dissolves and melts the resentments and energy strains that are ingrained in your memories and emotional worlds. The records of numerous unpleasant past experiences that have left wounds and scars inside your etheric (memory) bodies are the source of these pressures. At the smallest provocation, these wounds and scars exploded, releasing the venom of previous conflicts, misunderstandings, and enmities.

"Man knows not what he carries around with him buried deeply within that realm which science calls the **SUB-CONSCIOUS MIND**: that realm in which there are atrophied the memories of **EVERY EXPERIENCE IN EVERY EMBODIMENT** from the first day that the life stream **"fell from Grace"** up to the present moment.

Certain life streams, each of which holds these memories of past animosities between them, are repeatedly brought together by the Divine Plan presenting, repeatedly, new opportunities to **MAKE THINGS RIGHT.**

"**RIGHT NOW,** if there is any life stream in this Earth life with whom you are not in complete accord, **CONSCIOUSLY DRAW THE IMAGE OF THAT PERSON BEFORE YOUR MIND'S EYE** and let Me give you the pressure of **MY FEELING** of unconditional, loving forgiveness toward that one

Accepting this will free you from the drag of the energies from those previous errors.

12. CHAMUELL ARCHANGEL OF ADORATION:

The flame that you hold within the chalice of your heart is by its very nature adoration. By transferring this divine nature, you can return to your place of unity with God.

Oh, Immortal Flame of Life within these hearts! **Arise!** Let the song of thanksgiving, praise, and the immortal gratitude to the **Father-Mother God of light** I sing through the temple wherein thou dost dwell.

Oh, great and mighty flame within these hearts! Send forth thy rhythm of adoration to God! Send it forth with each heartbeat, waking, sleeping, day and night, until the perfume of spiritual adoration fills ones aura; until the essence of love divine forms a protective shell around each one; until the music and paean of praise is so tangible that even to enter the sphere of influence and touch the hem of the garment of each student, is to experience the bliss of Heaven. In a steady, joyful beat, you must adore your God with all your heart, soul, and entire being.

The Adoration Flame is an absolute basking in the Goodness of God. Adoration is a complete devotion to the goodness of life. It is the same relaxed devotion that you feel when you sit in the sunshine on a beautiful Spring day and absorb into yourself the goodness of the light of the mighty Sun. Adoration is the act of pouring out your life and all of your gratitude into the Sun's heart, your **I AM** Presence's heart, Saint Germain's heart, or the heart of any other godless person.

13. ORION, ELOHIM OF LOVE: Accept now, God's Love for you, and within it, your divinity, and your ability to express that love to all life with which you have contact, every day upon your individual paths. The best way to show God's love is to change yourself to improve the world!

Ask God's Love to fill your consciousness to overflowing, beloved ones, and open your heart and mind to the Third Ray. Allow the attribute of divine love to permeate all your thoughts and inspirations as you enjoy these rewards.

Love is not merely an emotional feeling you experience for others and life in general. It also must include the understanding of how to express that feeling faithfully, to bring forth the perfect manifestation you so deeply desire.

14. IN THE NAME OF THE PRESENCE OF GOD WHICH "I AM", I call to You, Beloved Paul, Lady Rowena, Chamuel, and Orion, and every Great Being and Power of Light who works on the Third Ray and with God's Pink Flame of Love, to **BLAZE (3) GOD'S PINK FLAME OF LOVE AND ADORATION** as Of a thousand suns into every part of my being and world, my loved ones, and every person, place, condition and thing; the Elemental Kingdom, birds, four-footed creatures, and every living thing upon our **EARTH RIGHT NOW**, and hold it there until all imprisoned life is set free by **GOD'S PINK FLAME OF LOVE. ¡I Thank You!**

15. Beloved Presence of God I AM in me; I love and adore you! *Oh, great and mighty flame within my own heart, blaze forth the pink flame of divine love until I AM the comforting presence to all life everywhere! I love, bless, and thank all the beings of light from the Third Ray, who assist me this day. As God's most holy name ... I*

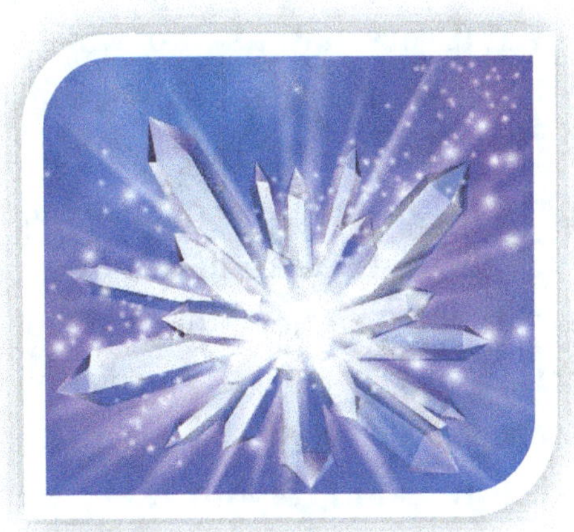

4.

WEDNESDAY

FOURTH RAY
WHITE FLAME
OF
PURITY RESURRECTION
AND ASCENSION

---

1. SERAPIS BEY, CHOHAN OF THE FOURTH RAY: Every day as you walk the path toward the full ascension into the light of your own, **I AM Presence**, receive and accept the magnificent feelings of joy and peace embodied in an of God's Gifts that you require to be happy in co-service with our Father-Mother God. Peace, harmony, and unity of life are provided by the Christ inside.

All life will respond to your every request to bring about the perfection that God wants for you once your consciousness has reached this higher level of awareness through the constant application of the sacred **Violet Fire** and the growing strength of the Ascension Flame. It is within this state of mastery that a true balance of energy is attained, and you are also able to perceive the need of others as they, too, progress upon this same spiritual path.

2. Dearly beloved Presence of God - "I AM" in me, and Beloved Holy Christ Self within my heart, I love and adore You! You know the **REASON** for my being, Through the energies of my world this day, **LET ME FULFILL IT!** See that I do not miss one opportunity; see that I never make a mistake of any kind; and let me avoid, **ABOVE ALL THINGS**, the sins **OMISSION!**

3. BELOVED CLAIRE, THE GREAT ELOHIM OF PURITY, says: "I AM" THE ELOHIM OF PURITY! "I AM" the living, breathing **PURITY** of the electron which lives in the center of the atoms of which your physical bodies are composed. "I AM" ALIVE in every cell of your body moving around the central core of every atom of your flesh. "I AM" WITH YOU ALWAYS! "I AM" YOUR LIFE! "I AM" the living, breathing Electronic Light of **PURITY** within your mental bodies so "I AM" the living, breathing Flame of Pure Light invoked by each of you into the great sea of your emotional world.

"I AM" the Electronic Light in each of your etheric garment's cells, onto which you have imprinted those impurity records, and "I AM" presently increasing my purity from within each of your four lower bodies' cells and atoms EXPANDING, EXPANDING, EXPANDING

The purification of this planet, everything on it, and everything in its atmosphere is my true nature. I **DECREE** that the **PURITY** within the heart of every one of your electrons shall now **EXPAND (3)** until that which appears as limitation can no longer imprison your life in discord, and thus the shadows **SHALL CEASE TO BE!"**

4. BELOVED ELOHIM OF PURITY, you have benefited me and all of humanity, and for that I love, bless, and thank You. I declare the **PURITY** of every electron in my aura, emotions, mind, etheric, and physical bodies. I seal myself and all of humanity in Your **Oval of Pure Blazing White Light**, which deflects those energy currents that slow the vibratory action of my inner bodies. shall now **EXPAND (3)** and that which is limitation and shadow in my world **SHALL BE NO MORE!**

5. GABRIEL, ARCHANGEL OF THE RESURRECTION: I AM here to announce to all the world with conviction, that not only does your Holy Christ This all-knowing, all-loving, all-powerful being of light lives inside you and is an essential part of you, dear ones!

It is time to acknowledge your duty and everything that goes along with it. In your hearts, the **Holy Christ** is a three-fold light being. You must be able to take on the role of the *Mother,* fostering and extending the divine idea of Christ for everyone on the planet. You must, as well, function as the *Father,* protecting and permitting nothing to bring harm to the

Mother or Child within each human heart. Finally, you must bring forth the Christ in such a way that others will understand that the example of the Christ is not something done by one human, but something that was given for all humankind! Silently ask yourself with every situation in your life: ***"How would the Master respond or react in each instance?"*** For in the very asking of this question you instantly reactivate and intensify the connection with your inner self and the answer will become clear.

6. BELOVED GABRIEL, ARCHANGEL OF THE RESURRECTION, says: *"Religion is not a matter of ceremony alone. It is a matter of **DAILY, HOURLY LIVING!** It comes down to simple common sense! It involves self-control, discipline, and introspection. It also involves the growth of love and gratitude for life itself and for the God who has given your life and kept you alive for millions of years in the hopes that he will use you to fulfil a destiny that no other individual can fulfil—some part of the vast cosmic tapestry that only your life-stream can fulfil."*

7. BELOVED GABRIEL, I love, bless, and, thank You for what You mean to me and to all mankind, **CHARGE** Your Cosmic pressure of Love into these - my decrees: **"I AM"** the **RESURRECTION AND THE LIFE** of all the **GOOD** in my life stream! **"I AM"** the **RESURRECTION**

AND THE LIFE of my eternal youth and beauty; perfect sight and hearing; limitless strength and energy; and my perfect health! of **"I AM"** the **RESURRECTION AND THE LIFE** my limitless supply. of money and every good and perfect thing! **"I AM"** the **RESURRECTION AND THE LIFE** of all Perfection in my world - and my Divine Plan fulfilled **RIGHT NOW!**

8. **BELOVED ASCENDED MASTER SERAPIS BEY,** Chohan of the Fourth Ray, says: **"The ASCENSION FLAME** is intelligent, beloved ones, and I have loved It long and lived It well. It can **ASCEND ANY CONDITION** in which you find yourself. It can ascend that condition from limitation into Harmony; from distress into peace; from poverty into opulence; from discord into perfection. It is one of the activities of **DIVINE ALCHEMY** which the student body, for the moat, part, have not thought about using.

If your life is burdened with difficulties; if your soul is burdened; if the people you work with are depressed, sometimes without your own depression; should you become aware of any economic downturns through your telecasts; then **CALL TO THE BROTHERHOOD OF LUXOR** to send the **ASCENSION FLAME** to bring into life and the ascendancy the buoyancy which resurrects the depression and brings it into a natural state of happiness and harmony.

The **Ascension Flame**, like the **Resurrection Flame,** is a most marvellous antidote for depression - individually and collectively."

9. ARCHANGEL OF RESTORATION: I AM the embodiment of the Heart Desire of our Father-Mother God, for the restoration of the beloved planet Earth and all life upon it, to complete unity, total atonement with God's First Cause-perfection for all things, and the restoration of this perfection is that for which I have been created! To the full glory of God, the truth of this beloved planet and every individual who lives on it shall be revealed once more!

The return of perfection on Earth will be ensured by your heart's yearning being united with your **Father-Mother God.** Keep the Earth's perfection and all her evolutions in the forefront of your mind. As I now direct a laser beam from my flame into your eager heart, accept and feel my love.

Through this act, we shall always be consciously connected. From this time forth we are **ONE** in love and **ONE** in service to the great Universal Source of all Life.

10. **BELOVED SERAPIS BEY**, I love, bless, and thank You for the Beloved Ascension Flame which is the **WAY BACK HOME** for me and for all humanity,

11. IN THE NAME OF MY OWN BELOVED PRESENCE OF GOD "I AM"; and that of all mankind, I call to You, Beloved Serapis Bey and the Brotherhood at Luxor to **KEEP THE ASCENSION FLAME BLAZING (3)** through my feelings, my mind, my etheric body, my physical body, my home, my business, and all my affairs.

Allow its stimulating action to Raise everything in my universe to forever maintained love, happiness, opulence, victory, and perfection. When my earthly mission is over, guide me into the victory of my ascension.

Keep **THE ASCENSION FLAME BLAZING (3)** through the **BUSINESS WORLD** and the minds and feelings of every part of life evolving on the planet Earth to more quickly bring Perfection.

¡I Thank You!

12. CLAIRE, ELOHIM OF PURITY:
I AM the Flame of Cosmic Christ Purity, the natural activity of your own life.

I AM alive in every cell of your body, moving around the central core of every atom of your flesh.

I AM your life!

I AM the living breathing electronic light of purity within your mental bodies, waiting now to be released to manifest the perfection of your divine conception.

I AM the living, breathing, flame of pure white light, invoked by each one of you into the great sea of your emotional world, awaiting release to again manifest perfection.

I AM the pure electronic light within every cell of your etheric garment, upon which you have impressed those records of impurity.

I AM now expanding my purity from within every cell and atom of your four lower vehicles expanding, expanding, and expanding my true nature which is the purification of this Earth; all that is in the Earth; on it, or in its atmosphere.

I AM the guardian of the Immaculate Concept for this sweet planet Earth, as well as for this entire universe.

Dearly beloved **Presence of God I AM** in me; I love and adore you. You know the reason for my being, through the energies of my world this day, let me fulfil.

I love, bless, and thank all the beings of light from the Fourth Ray, who assist me this day. As God's most holy name ... **I AM.**

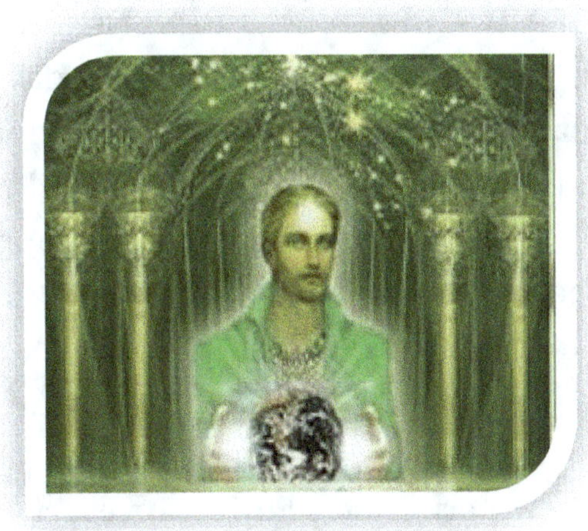

5.

THURSDAY
FIFTH RAY GREEN FLAME
OF
TRUTH HEALING
CONSECRATION
CONCENTRATION

---

1. DEARLY BELOVED PRESENCE OF GOD "I AM" in me, I consecrate my life this day to the service of God-Good to let only Perfection take thought in my brain; that my feelings will remain calm and loving, kindly, helpful, and happy; my eyes to see Perfection; my ears to hear Perfection; my lips to speak only Perfection; my hands to bless and heal; my feet to be messengers of Good; my body strong and willing to be a helpful instrument to carry God's Perfection everywhere.

2. BELOVED HILARION, CHOHAN OF THE FIFTH RAY, says: *"God's Presence would flow through a person on the return currents as the fullness of everything he could desire if he first understood the power of sustained attention, then, through self-conscious endeavour, wrest the attention away from the many pulls of the appearance world and anchor that attention on the **PRESENCE OF GOD."***

*"Where your attention is, there you are; what your attention is upon - that you **BECOME!"*** declared the Ascended Master Saint Germain on several occasions. The Universe is filled with radiation and the love and mercy of God, yet I am completely ignorant of it.

The LEVER for the man who wishes to proceed in self-conscious action is the controlled power of his attention, yet both the just and the unjust are impacted by this outpouring of **God's forgiveness."**

3. HILARION, CHOHAN OF THE FIFTH RAY: The first step is the preparation of your own chalice of consciousness for service with the Octaves of Light. The Cosmic Ray of Truth and the Violet Transmuting Flame must be invoked after summoning the protection of the First Ray.

Anything that prevents you from becoming fully united with your higher bodies will be made visible to your outer consciousness by the Ray of Truth. After that, the Violet Flames transform these causes and cores, clearing your own chalice of any uncertainty or other impediment that might be tying your spiritual consciousness to the human one.

Once these preparatory steps have been taken, you are ready to offer your individual chalice of consciousness to your **I AM Presence.**

As you progress in the service of self-healing, your body elemental will mirror that which you have changed in your etheric body through your conscious effort and full cooperation. These beloved ones, begins the process of re-unifying your four lower vehicles; and as you stabilize and remain in this state, with crystal I need clear feelings thoughts, memories, actions and words, your natural state of being is restored.

At that moment, the extension of your divine pattern of expression starts to spread outward, providing all your human family members with an example that they will want to follow. Right now, in the realm of form, you will be the outward manifestation of perfect health and harmony.

4. BELOVED HILARION, I appreciate, love, and thank you for helping me and all of humanity. Give me your love, your comprehension of the cosmic law's exactness, and the sense of dedicated service to both God and humanity. **CHARGE** me with **YOUR MOMENTUM** of presenting the Truth to humanity so that all who hear will accept it. **I THANK YOU!**

5. BELOVED RAPHAEL,

"Consecrate yourselves every day," encourages the Archangel of Healing and Consecration. You know where **"I AM"** is if you perceive iniquity, and you just say in silence, **"FATHER, FORGIVE ME FOR BREAKING YOUR LAW OF LOVE;** and, Beloved Raphael, consecrate my eyes to see only Perfection!"

If you listen to gossip or discord; if your hands are impatient in gesture and you release anger; if your lips and tongue, use sharp words, say: **"Father, forgive me for the misuse of Your energy!** What if you do have to repeat it? Paderewski did not suddenly become a great musician!

Those live streamers who do not want to get back up and try again are the only ones in danger. I will re-consecrate any member of your vehicles twenty-four times an hour if You will ask Me, and you require it! I do not mind - **IT IS MY REASON FOR BEING!"**

6. RAPHAEL, ARCHANGEL OF HEALING AND CONSECRATION: I offer you my Cup of Consecration, that you may renew your vows made at inner levels, to be the healers and teachers of the New Age. Remember, as you drink from this cup, the essence of my flame flows through your entire being and encompasses your aura.

I give you the courage and strength you need when this happens, and you will have it going ahead. You can extract enough wonderful things to last you a lifetime from the Realms of Light. You are our nope, our love, and our healing manifest on the Earth ... right here, right now and forever sustained.

When consecration is coupled with dedication, it is a true feeling that will help you in all you do. When one is resolute, you are accepting and offering your service to a lofty ideal. When you dwell within the Christ; when you know **I AM** the **DOER,** the **DOING,** and the **DEED,** then you are doing God's Way. Remain centred, dear children, for you have come a far way on the path, or else you would not be here.

7. BELOVED RAPHAEL, I love, bless, and thank You for all that You have done for me and for all humankind. Seal us in Your Flame of Consecration and Perfection and help me to be conscious ***ONLY of PERFECTION, I THINK PERFECTION! I FEEL PERFECTION! I SEE PERFECTION! I HEAR PERFECTION! I SPEAK PERFECTION! "I AM" and I MANIFEST ONLYPERFECTION THIS DAY!***

8. BELOVED VISTA. (Cyclopean) Elohim of Concentration, Music, and the All- Seeing Eye of God to our Earth, says: ***"What can be accomplished on Earth even in mundane activities of your daily living without CONCENTRATION?*** If there is no Concentration, there is only mediocrity; only the bare surface is scratched. People who choose to stand out from the crowd choose one aspect of life and develop it to a high degree, choosing to succeed in at least one area of expression.

According to the **CONCENTRATION OF THOSE ENERGIES** is their development - is their mastery - is their efficacy. *"It is Law - actual scientific Law -* that what you begin **CAN BE ACCOMPLISHED** when it is an agreement with God's Plan of Perfection - whether it be healing, precipitation, financial freedom, eternal youth, or the restoration of a limb, **IT CAN BE DONE**, but the 'stick-to-it liveness of My Ray is required to produce these results!"

9. BELOVED VISTA, I love, bless, and thank You for Your great service to our Earth. **CHARGE** me with Your Power of **CONCENTRATION** and to become Master here and now. **I THANK YOU!**

10. ELOHIM VISTA, THE ALL-SEEING EYE OF GOD: I AM dedicated to expanding the power of concentration into all that is of the light, until all humankind can realize their fullest potential which is total unity with the **PRESENCE OF GOD I AM** within. The ability to focus is a gift that you must use in all facets of your life until you have used your love and concentration skills to change everything in your expression from human to divine.

Everyone has a being, but only a select few are aware of its true nature; this is what the ability to focus must be used to uncover. You were made in the image and likeness of the Highest Living God, which is the truth about you.

The purpose of the inner eye is to lift your gaze toward the Presence of **God I AM** for every instruction. When this is fully understood, you will take great care to permit your vision, inner or outer, to rest only upon conditions. that you wish to encounter, for manifest they shall!

11. ATHENA, SPIRIT OF TRUTH: *I AM the Way, I AM the Truth, and I AM the Life*. For you to live a truly spiritual life, you must experience clearing away every error, every desire, every prejudice, and every ha bit that stands in your path. The light within you will lead you home only once you have cleaned this away.

Accepting the truth frequently means letting go of long-held beliefs, even some that you hold dear. Both the seeker and the finding are typically forced to make new mental modifications when they accept the truth. Although the truth is **"simple"**, it is not always **"easy"**. Do not allow old concepts and old ways to keep you from the truth. Each time you call for light to be brought into any situation, you are making a real contribution to all life on Earth.

Dearly beloved **Presence of God I AM** in me; I consecrate my life this day to the service of God. Let me on see, feel, think, and conduct God s Perfection. I love, bless, and thank all the beings of light from the Fifth Ray, who assist me this day. As God's most holy name ... **I AM.**

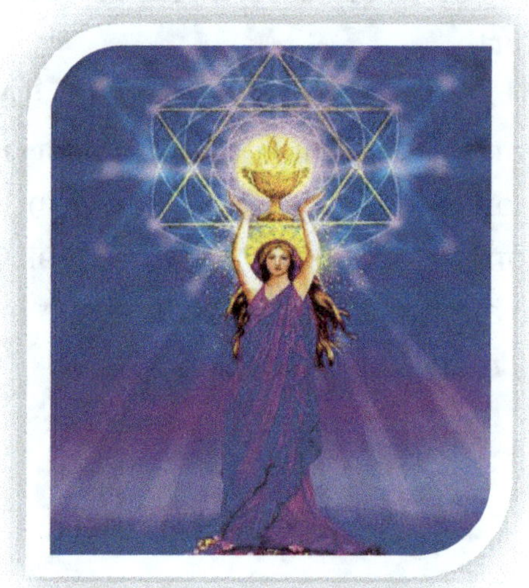

6.

FRIDAY
SIXTH RAY GOLD AND RUBY
FLAMES
OF
PEACE HEALING GRACE
MINISTRATION

---

1. **PRESENCE OF GOD - "I AM"** in me, I love and adore You, pour forth through me this day Your Pink and Gold Flames to bless every cell of my physical body and all the Powers of Nature that serve me so well. May all who touch the hem of my garment' feel Your Love, Your Peace, and Your Perfection, for **"I AM" THE PRESENCE OF BLESSING; AND I BLESS EVERYONE AND EVERYTHING I CONTACT THIS DAY!**

2. **JOHN, THE BELOVED, CHOHAN OF SIXTH RAY:**

I AM called Beloved because I know that I AM Beloved of God. What is true for me, is also true for you.

I AM one who reveals the truth of God's Love for you, and for all life.

I AM part of the activity of the Cosmic Holy Spirit, because I always reveal the love nature of the Father-Mother God.

*My beloved ones, you must embrace your true divinity. **"Let go and let God BE God in and through you",** for this is your true self, the divine archetype, who is now, ever has been, and ever shall be!* However, by letting go and letting God, you are releasing your human will to the thoughts, feelings, actions, and reactions of Christ Consciousness within.

This is the part that is up to you and needs to be completed using your free will and outer consciousness. The heavenly gift that separates divine consciousness from human consciousness is free will. This is a treasured gift. The outcome of the planet that will be created depends on whether your divine consciousness or your human awareness uses it. This is the key which you may use to allow the Kingdom of Heaven to manifest upon the Earth. This is the "letting go", beloved ones.

3. URIEL, ARCHANGEL OF MINISTRATION, PEACE, AND GRACE:
Wherever the name of God is invoked, silently or audibly, there I AM with the fullness of the love, the blessings, the healing, the faith, and the power of the Almighty. I say to your consciousness, to your minds and to your bodies, *"In the name of the One Mighty God, peace be unto you! Let it enter NOW into every cell and fibber of your being as you relax in the knowledge that you are immersed in the Presence of the Almighty!"*

4. DONNA GRACE, ARCHAII OF THE SIXTH RAY: Remember, beloved ones, that by the Grace of God, you descended to this Earth You will stay in a state of grace. And one day you shall sore back into the **Heart of our Father-Mother God**

through the Gift of Grace! Every individual is on a spiritual quest or heavenly trip that will eventually bring them full circle and bring them back to our Father-Mother God at all levels of consciousness.

5. BELOVED JESUS, FORMER CHOHAN OF THE SIXTH RAY, says: *"Unless he learns to consciously quiet the energies of his own world, the demands placed on the time, energy, attention, and service of the chela who is involved in a spiritual endeavour will be a major obstacle to his personal growth. This will allow his own "I AM" Presence and the Di vine Beings who are so willing to help him to provide him with new strength, faith, and power.*

*I know this from My own experience. During My Ministry, as today, the world and its people require so much assistance. There is a tendency to **RUSH FORTH** to serve without the necessary period of re-fuelling at the Cosmic Fount.*

*You will recall from some of my experiences that I frequently prayed in the hills. No chela can be of lasting service to the spiritual work at hand unless he understands the necessity of taking time - **UNDIVIDED** - from the world (which you will always) have with you} to enter the **SILENCE** and draw the necessary strength and sanctity* *from the Source of **ALL GOOD**. This he can then dispense in poise, dignity, and loving solicitude for his fellowman."*

6. BELOVED JESUS, I love, bless, and thank You for all You mean to me and to all humanity. **CHARGE** me with the **Ascended Jesus Christ Consciousness and Love,** and the Power to do the things that You have done.

7. JOHN, THE BELOVED, NOW THE CHOHAN OF THE SIXTH RAY, says: "You begin training your own four lower vehicles first when you join the Great White Brotherhood.

Since you are the conduit for the energies of light and love, it is understood that your own four vehicles must be in some sort of order for you to assist others. However, keep in mind that ten billion spirits will be following you when you receive such an instruction and beg for grace to endure it.

So don't leave one pitfall of which you are cognizant into which they unwittingly in their desire to serve life might fall; one mis- interpretation of a word, a sentence, which might be utilized as license instead of freedom, for this is a Pact between Heaven and Earth made by you and your Maker.

8. JOHN, THE BELOVED, I love, bless, and thank you for your great service to the Earth. Keep us sealed in the Power of the Sixth Ray, that heals, loves, and blesses all **Life FREE!**

9. BELOVED URIEL, ARCHANGEL OF MINISTRATION, says:

*"The Ministering Angel has to WILL Himself to serve ONE livestream. There is one for everyone who belongs to the human race, every laggard from other systems, and every **Guardian Spirit,** a particular and specific **Ministering Angel** who volunteers to be that Protecting Presence in, through and around that life stream for so long as he or she chooses to remain on the Earth or part of its evolution.*

*That being is often referred to as the **Guardian Angel.** How would you like to work with just **ONE** person for countless millions of years? Your Guardian Angel does not even attend a Retreat when it is active if the livestream He is guarding does not go! Think on that! There is no comparable instance of incarceration through love. According to the law, the ministering angel must accompany everyone around, delivering a light beam into the consciousness a bit higher at every chance the thought that they will seek a little higher."*

10. BELOVED URIEL, I love, bless, and thank You and my **MINISTERING ANGEL** for Your selfless service to me through aeons of time. *Help me to help my Angel keep me steadily on the Path of Purity, Harmony, and Happiness.*

11. TRANQUILLITY, ELOHIM OF PEACE: You can experience I AM Consciousness and be at one with all life Be I AM at all times, and you will be a PEACE COM MANDI NG PRESENCE, radiating the quality of peace with every thought, word or deed ... precipitating at all times with every breath the spirit of the one universal feeling of I AM. Since peace is so important to upholding the decree of cosmic law, now is the moment to be I AM and to spread this virtue. Knowing that serenity is your best defence, you will experience your consciousness growing and engulfing the cosmos in the oneness of being. Affirm within your mind, I **AM A** PEACE **COMMANDING** PRESENCE, and in the oneness of I AM, PEACE SHALL MANIFEST. LADY NADA, former Chohan of the **Sixth Ray:** Love is the power that holds the universe together. It is the love emanating from the Father-Mother God to each of Earth's children that sets all constructive ideas into motion. Seeing the gift of love at work in your life, all around you, and within you is the most powerful and reliable evidence you will ever have. You must be focused on this unadulterated, divine level always.

12. BELOVED TRANQUILITY, THE GREAT ELOHIM OF PEACE, says: "I AM" the **ELOHIM OF MINISTRATION AND PEACE!** You who have given your interest and your life to the activities of the Seventh Ray, represented by Our Beloved Ascended Master Saint Germain, are slowly, but surely, emerging from the mire of human creation and limitation, We are endeavouring to build a great foundation for this World Movement; trying to make of each of you a mighty pillar with Of the Violet Fire.

But I can tell you here and now that unless you hold **UN INTERRUPTED PEACE** as separate individuals and collective units - no matter how perfectly you build - you would have but ash in the end as long as there was still within the consciousness of any worker the disintegrating radiation of the **'SEVEN MORTAL SINS** *(lust and passion, anger, malice, hatred, fear, greed, gluttony, covetousness, lethargy and laziness, envy, pride and arrogance)* and all their ramifications.

"Peace is not a negative quality, it is the most **POSITIVE** and most concentrated activity of

Power, how much Power of control does it require for you to **HOLD YOUR PEACE.**

TO REMAIN ABSOLUTELY POISED AND MASTER OF EVERY SITUATION REGARDLESS OF THE AGGRAVATION IN THE MIDST OF YOUR IMMEDIATE FAMILY, BUSINESS AND WORLD AT LARGE?"

13. ENCOURAGEMENT IS A SPECIAL FACET OF DIVINE LOVE.

Encouraging someone entails giving them the strength of your faith in their potential to succeed in whatever their work may be, as well as a spirit of courage. The goal is the full realisation of Saint Germain's Permanent Golden Age, and it is imperative that all efforts be united for the good of the planet. Each chela and light worker must live and work in harmony and unity for this to become a manifest reality. You must know that whatever is going on around you at any time is a manifestation of the Perfection of God.

14. BELOVED PRESENCE OF GOD - "I AM"

in me and in all humanity. Beloved Jesus, Nada, Uriel, my own Ministering Angel, and Great Elohim of Peace, I love, bless, and thank You in the name of all humankind for Your service to our Earth for so long.

BLAZE {3} YOUR COSMIC FLAMES OF LOVE, GRACE, MINISTRATION, HEALING AND PEACE INTO ME AND LET THEM RADIATE THROUGH ME TO BLESS AND HELP HARMONIZE EVERY PART OF LIFE I CONTACT. Great Elohim of Peace, enfold all my don constructive efforts in Your great Flame of Love and Peace.

BLAZE YOUR FLAME OF PEACE (3) as of a thousand suns into the brain and feelings of every living thing on our Earth and everyone who will come here in the future - and hold it sustained until **PEACE ON EARTH -- GOOD WILL TO ALL LIFE IS A LIVING REALITY TO BE FOREVER SUSTAINED AND EVER-EXPANDING.** We Thank You.

15. Blessed Presence of God I AM in me; I love and adore you. Pour forth through me this day your pink and gold flames to bless everyone and everything I contact this day I love, bless, and thank all the beings of light from the Sixth Ray, who assist me this day. As God's most holy name **... I AM.**

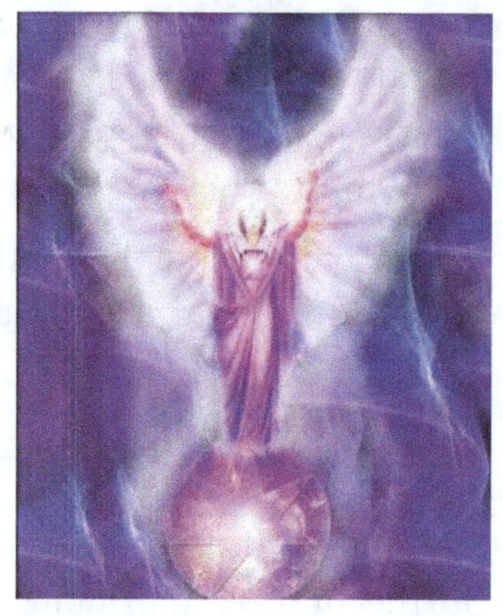

7.

SATURDAY

SEVENTH RAY VIOLET0 FIRE
OF
MERCY COMPASSION
INVOCATION TRANSMUTATION
AND FREEDOM

---

1. SAINT GERMAIN, CHOHAN OF EVE NTH RAY: Lasting balance can only be attained within the heart of the great, Great, Silence. Only then will you be able to find the wisdom, love, and strength required to raise your Threefold Flame's frequency into harmony with God. You may achieve the ideal harmony and balance you desire as you let your inner Christ Consciousness carry you into the centre of your Presence! Your Spirit transforms into a higher vibratory action in this way, advancing to embrace and bless all existence. Make a conscious effort to spend time in the Great Silence every day.

As the radiance of Violet Fire intensifies and expands around you, your world of expression increases, and you are enfolded in the flame of transmutation. Have faith in the Violet Fire, and it will provide you with the answer. Remember, you are an integral part of your **I AM Presence**, and through the power of your attention, you can reach the inner most treasures of your causal body. The divinity within you validates the interconnectedness of all life and bestows blessings onto everyone else! You can be sure that I am pulled to your heart and you to mine as the **Violet Fire** becomes a conscious and continuous emanation from your heart centre. Bringing the infinite number of livestreams with their various levels of consciousness that have chosen Earth as their home together into a single, harmonious global activity is the main challenge in creating this New Age. Each livestream is special and must perform their assigned task in unity and love to enhance the glory of the others. Concern yourselves only with the divine will of our *Father Mother God.*

2. Dearly Beloved Presence of God - "I AM" in me; **TODAY "I AM" RENEWED! TODAY "I AM" ALIVE** with that primal pure majestic life given to me of the Father. For yesterday's life misused, **I CALL ON THE LAW OF FORGIVENESS** and accept the most powerful activity of the Transmuting Violet Fire, for **TODAY,** within my magic Mantle of Light **- MY RING - PASS NOT OF FLAME,** I have the gifts of God's Life unsullied - pure - clean.

Today **I MAY BECOME;** today **I SHALL BECOME** that which God intends -- **MY HOLY CHRIST SELF IN ACTION'** for **"I AM" THE CHRIST CONSCIOUSNESS (3)** now made manifest and eternally sustained. Keep me **SEALED** in a Pillar of Violet Fire that transcends all human creation in, through, and around me, or that which is returning for redemption, until **"I AM",** wholly ascended and free!

3.   **BELOVED ASCENDED MASTER SAINT GER- MAIN,** Chohan of the Seventh Ray, and the Master in charge of the Earth and its evolutions for the next two thousand years, says: "Take time to be holy! **LEARN,** I ask of you, to **GET STILL** even when there is no apparent emergency! **PRACTICE** just **STILLING** your thought processes from racing; just stopping your etheric memories from resuscitating all of the discords; just stopping the restless motion of your physical body; and then if you can, without making your mental body immediately start working again, just turn quietly **TO ONE BEING** and tune in until you can anchor yourself in **PEACE. ONE SUCH PERSON** could save a city!

"**I AM**" **DETERMINED** that the realization and the science of the use of the Violet Fire shall find anchorage in some unaccented being as an **ABSOLUTE IRREFUTABLE SCIENTIFIC MANIFESTATION** --- which cannot be denied!

"**I AM**" more eager for you to learn to use this Violet Fire than you will ever be because YOU **HAVE TO BE MYSELF** in the world of form --as I, by Cosmic Law, must remain behind the veil. *"You who are My friends - ACCEPT ME!"*

Let Me walk the Earth through you; let Me help you with this Divine Alchemy, come to the Violet Fire Temples at night and I will sit with you and explain over and over the science and Divine Alchemy of this Violet Fire.

KNOW that there is a place for you in the Home and Heart of Saint Germain!"

4. BELOVED ZADKIEL, ARCHANGEL OF INVOCATION AND TRANSMUTATION, says: "Do you know that the LIFE within an **UNKIND WORD** comes to you to be **REDEEMED AND SET FREE?** The life within an unkind look or gesture comes to you - a Priest or Priestess of the Order of Zadkiel, you might **BLESS IT FREE!"**

Let us avoid personalising energy, which is found in your everyday experiences and thoughts. If circumstances are such that energy qualified with discord appears within the scope of your aura, do not resist against it or feel unfairly treated. This is because there are not many foci in this unaccented Octave that know how to raise or redeem it; to purify it; to set it free, *"Where there is a focus of the Sacred Fire, where there is a livestreams who has a knowledge of the Violet Flame; there that energy has an opportunity of being redeemed and returned to the Universal First Cause."*

Oh, what joy to move in the Universe freeing energy; loving it free; and standing in the serene mastery of your own Godhood I words that are spoken even lightly (jokingly) to or ·about another part of life **WHICH DO NOT BLESS IT** are, therefore, a malediction. I ask that all life streams be released from the recoil of such mistakes!"

5. **ARCTURUS, ELOHIM OF INVOCATION, RHYTHM, AND FREEDOM:** My divine quality of rhythm is a very necessary part in the process of mastering the use of the Violet Fire. The Violet Fire will immediately begin to provide the service of increasing the vibration of energy upon your request and visualisation, transforming its quality to perfection. You must learn to use it so well that it becomes an integral part of your being.

6. **BELOVED ARCTURUS, ELOHIM OF INVOCATION, RHYTHM, AND FREEDOM,** says: "I AM" the Elohim of **INVOCATION and RHYTHM** who brings to you and all life, using the Violet Fire, **INFINITE FREEDOM** - when you desire it enough! **"I AM"** He who answers the call" of the heartbeat of any individual when that heart deeply and sincerely, from within itself, desires to release life which has become bound giving it **FREEDOM** from disease, from lack, from fear and limitation of every kind and description.

Within that life itself is the **FULNESS OF ALMIGHTY GOD!** "Today I urge you, with all the in- tensity and pressure of My Being, to **DEVELOP YOUR LIFE**; develop the qualities of Perfection which are within it. Call forth what you wish from the Heart of that Life which flows from the Universe, and call to Me if you wish to release into the outer manifestation from within your own life whatever powers, qualities, gifts and activities are required to perfect your own individual world and that of your fellowman.

Wherever there is **ONE LIFESTREAM** who desires **FREEDOM**, and in constant **RHYTHM**, invokes and commands it, **THERE I SHALL BE** to give that one assistance until that **FREEDOM IS PHYSICALLY MANIFEST!"**

7. ZADKIEL, ARCHANGEL OF INVOCATION AND TRANSMUTATION:

Those who have gained a significant degree of spiritual freedom know there is a deep responsibility involved. True freedom is a gift that requires maintenance and upkeep and should always be treasured. The Threefold Flame in your heart is combined with the strength and activity of transformation. You possess the power because God has anchored it in you in the magnificent chalice of your heart. Because the words of the Ascended Host of Light have been continually revealed to you by cosmic law, you possess wisdom. God loves you because you are here.

Every day, engage in a rhythmic action that allows the Violet Fire to burn brightly in your etheric, mental, emotional, and physical bodies. Pay particular attention to the structure and feeling world of your brain and give it instructions to transform any difficult or unforgiving emotions.

Breathe in deeply, experience the peace and comfort of my liquid light and life substance entering your aura, cleansing, and purifying it. You are now able to feel how loved by God you are and how you can love others, just as God loves you. Breathe in the pure essence of our Father-Mother God, so you can continue your onward and upward path toward your ascension in the light.

8. LADY KWAN YIN, SPIRIT OF MERCY AND COMPASSION: The impetus of the Seventh Ray exerts its influence on each one, at their own level of evolution. The same stimulus elicits distinct reactions as spiritual consciousness grows. Your four lower vehicles' vibration is increasing at a rate that could make you uncomfortable and show up as unbalance of some kind.

Situations in both personal and communal settings may call for more tolerance, love, and understanding than you now believe you possess. Give yourself more time to relax during this procedure so that your body can assimilate our lessons.

Give yourself time to connect the inner teachings with your physical experiences and situations. Be confident that all will become clear to you at the right time.

9.   BELOVED ASCENDED MASTER SAINT GERMAIN, BELOVED ZADKIEL, BELOVED ARCTURUS AND ALL who serve on the Seventh Ray, I love, bless, and thank You for Your mighty service to me and to all humankind.

IN THE NAME OF THE PRESENCE OF GOD WHICH "I AM", and by the magnetic power of the Sacred Fire vested in me as a Priest (Priestess) of the Order of Zadkiel,

I make this call: ***ANGELS OF' THE VIOLET FIRE (3) COME (3)*** and keep the ***VIOLET FIRE OF FREEDOM'S LOVE BLAZING (3)***

- through my aura and feelings.

- my brain and mental world.

- my etheric body.

- every cell of my physical body.

- my home, my family

- business,

- finances and affairs; and **DO THAT FOR EVERY PART OF LIFE ON THE PLANET UNTIL ALL HUMAN CREATION THERE,** its cause and core is dissolved and transmuted into Purity and Perfection, and our Earth is truly **FREEDOM'S HOLY STAR!**

I thank you for the answer to this - my Heart's Call-for **THE VIOLET FIRE OF FREEDOM'S LOVE NEVER FAILS (3) TO PRODUCE PURITY AND PERFECTION;** and **"I AM" THAT VIOLET FIRE!**

Mercy is more kindness than justice requires. It is more kindness than can be claimed by merit or service ... and forgiveness. Where you see distress of mind and body ... stop for a moment and consciously forgive the misuse of energy that created such an appearance and set it free.

10. BELOVED ASCENDED MASTER SAINT GERMAIN and **BELOVED GODDESS OF OPPORTUNITY:** I pledge my **LIFE,** my **LIGHT,** and my **LOVE** to You by endeavouring to release the momentums of Perfection in my life- stream to assist You, in bringing **FREEDOM TO EVERY PART OF LIFE** on our dear planet Earth as quickly as possible. **SO, BE IT!**

Beloved Presence of God I AM in me, keep me sealed in a pillar of violet fire that transcends all human creation in, through and around me, until I AM ascended and free! I love, bless, and thank all the beings of light from the Seventh Ray, who assist me this day. As God's most holy name ... I AM.

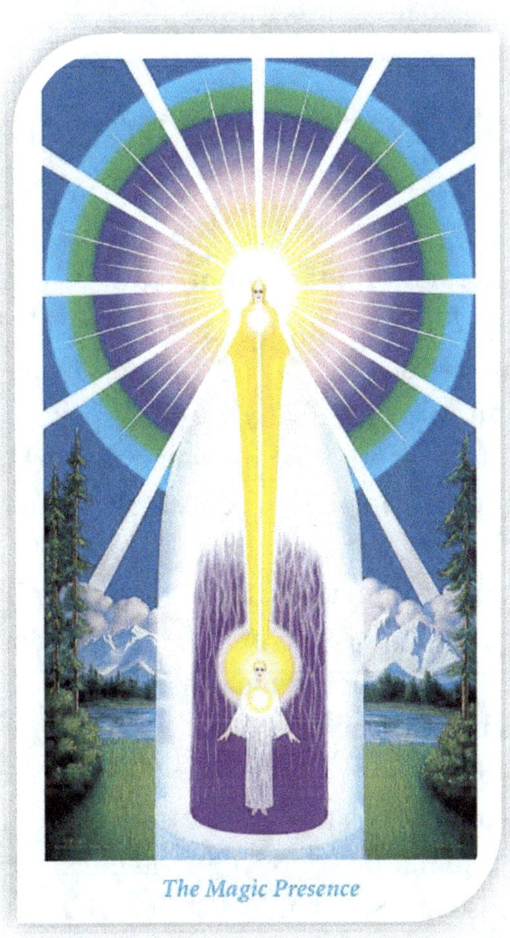

The Magic Presence

PRIMARY INSTRUCTION

PART 1

EXPLANATION OF THE HOLY TRINITY

The First Commandment says: *"Thou shall have NO OTHER GODS before Me"!* Therefore, we call your attention first to your own great individualized God Presence - "I AM" which stands above and enfolds you, and which is represented in the picture of the Holy Trinity

In the beginning, God sent forth this enormous, wonderful God Being. All the attributes and powers of the Father God are contained in this electronic presence, which is as bright as the midday sun.

The "Silver Cord" that enters the body through the pineal gland at the top of the skull and anchors a miniature of Itself in the physical heart is how this God Self sends a stream of Electronic Essence into the physical form.

It is LIFE that makes the heartbeat, allows the lungs to breathe, and gives you the strength to walk down the street, lift your hand, and conduct all of life's activities.

This Miniature of God in each heart makes every man, woman, and child a God or Goddess in embryo. Therefore, within everyone is the same power that enabled Jesus to perform the many manifestations of Perfection.

The object of every true religion down through the ages has been to assist the seeking soul to find this GOD WITHIN and loose the God Powers locked there; to allow the Flame within the heart to expand until Its Light and Perfection fills the individual's being and enabled him to 'graduate' into a higher sphere of service in the Victory of the Ascension and thus fulfil the words of Jesus: "The things I do, all men shall do!"

The Name of this Individualized God Presence is "I AM" - the Name of God as He gave it to Moses. The words "I AM" arc the great CREATIVE WORDS of Life. They draw into manifestation whatever follows them - whether it be constructive or otherwise. Jesus used these words in all His important statements, viz. ***"I AM" the Resurrection and the Life; "I AM" the Way, the Truth, and the Life';" 'I AM' the Open Door which no man can shut!"***

His most potent declaration was the first one, which allowed Him to record His resurrection and ascension as proof of the veracity of His teachings.

If it is difficult to accept the fact that you do have this glorious **"I AM"** Presence enfolding you, think quietly upon it when you are alone. It is the Secret of the Ages which all the Sages throughout history have known. Earnestly ask your own God Self - your own "I AM" - to assist you in knowing and accepting the Truth whenever it is presented to you.

Here is a rough example that can help you understand what we are attempting to convey. If you imagine a massive water tank with billions of faucets beneath it, and a stream of water streaming out of each faucet, you will see billions of streams of water, each is distinct but all originating from the same central source—the tank.

Now if you will think of that tank as Almighty God, and each stream of water a stream of Life - all separate, yet all coming from the One God, it may assist you in understanding that which we are trying to explain. When he possesses the latent ability to do and achieve anything he wants, man is always looking outside of himself for guidance, love, supply, and healing. The 'Bluebird' narrative serves as a good example of this.

As you may recall, the two kids in the picture were unhappy with their own modest home and resolved to search outside for the Bluebird of Happiness.

They looked everywhere for it, in the past, in the future, and in luxury·. When they could not find it there, they went back to their tiny house, completely disheartened, and THERE, in their own kitchen, was the Bluebird they had been looking for.

When man stops looking outside of himself and starts looking within his own heart, he, too, will find not only the Bluebird of Happiness, but all that he has ever craved - for so long!

The Ascended Masters, through ***THE BRIDGE TO SPIRITUAL FREEDOM TEACHINGS,*** are turning humankind, repeatedly, back to this **God Power - "I AM"** - within their hearts. Now they are again turning to that **" I AM"** for advice, for Love, for Illumination, for Healing, or whatever it is they desire.

"Seek you first the Kingdom of God, and then truly all things shall be added!" According to the Ascended Master Jesus, *"I meant to point man to the WAY by which he, too, might partake of the natural God Powers and Qualities that are within his own life when I repeatedly referred to 'the Father within' as the Power that accomplished all the seemingly miraculous manifestations during My Ministry."*

Every person eventually must connect with the God Presence that is his own heartbeat. Before a man may become a Representative of the Father to his fellow humans through his own nature, he must first undergo this mystic experience.

To find God within another is a cause for rejoicing in the unfoldment of that one's own God Flame; but to find God WITHIN ONESELF is the purpose for embodiment and the only way Home again into the natural estate of Blessedness, Peace and Power which such God awareness brings.

You might ask now why these imperfections are in your world if you are a part of God with the **"I AM"** Presence enfolding you and beating your heart. Because of God's Gift to you of free will! You have the power to create even as God has, and you are given freedom to CHOOSE what you wish to create - what qualities you desire to place upon your life which comes to you pure and perfect.

You become the custodian of that life when it comes to you, therefore you will eventually have to account for how you have used it. The Circle of Colours, sometimes referred to as the Causal Body, contains all your existence that has been qualified by your thoughts and feelings with positive attributes.

All the life energy upon which you have placed something less than Perfection, is around the physical form and is the pressure of discord which you feel.

The **VIOLET TRANSMUTING FLAME** is the Divine Tool provided by Life by which this human creation (or sins) can be dissolved and transmuted back into Perfection in a painless way. It is especially about this **VIOLET TRANSMUTING FLAME** that we wish to talk in this Lesson.

THE LAW OF THE CIRCLE

The Law of the Circle is one of God's great Universal Laws and is sometimes referred to as the Law of Cause and Effect, or *'what you sow, you reap!'*.

You are 'home' to that life and energy, so once it has arrived at its destination, it starts its journey back 'home', accumulating more of that specific quality or vibration with which it was initially charged. What you put upon your thoughts, feelings, words, and actions first passes through your own being and world before going out to the person, place, condition, or thing to which it is directed.

Therefore, you receive back into your world that which you sent forth - amplified - whether it was constructive or destructive. If you criticize, you will be criticized; if you hurt someone, you will be hurt; if you are unkind and unjust, harshness and injustice will come back to you.

Before you may be free from the **EFFECTS** of these established **CAUSES,** you must balance and modify them. Planting grain yields corn: planting disharmony yields discord; planting flowers yields flowers; and planting love, kindness, and constructive causes yields the same results in effects.

How can intelligent individuals think they can receive good health, love, supply, happiness, and all the other positive aspects of life while yet sending out or "planting" criticism, annoyance, unkindness, impurity, and all other harmful qualities?

The entire world is currently experiencing chaos, confusion, and distress of all kinds because of the destructive qualities that have been unleashed by the human mind, including hate, greed, selfishness, cruelty, and everything else.

When YOUR life injures some other part of life through thoughts, feeling, spoken word or deed, a **CAUSE** or debt of energy is set up which sometime, somewhere, must be met and **PAID!**

Many times, the person you wronged (or the person who wronged you) dies before the debt is paid off. For this reason, it is necessary to provide a future opportunity for the parties to meet again, through normal circumstances, and try to balance and harmonise the debt by providing a service to the person who was harmed.

These adjustments can be and often are made by the bringing together of such livestreams in a future embodiment in which they may learn to work together harmoniously.

THE LAW OF RE-EMBODIMENT

Re-embodiment is a **TRUTH,** and the only logical explanation for the many apparent injustices which can be seen around us.

You may be certain that there is no mistake, but that everyone is dealing with the consequences of past causes that were established somewhere in the past and of which they have no memory, when you see good, constructive people going through extremely trying times while others who do not seem to be living in such a constructive manner seem to be enjoying all the good things in life.

What they go through in the future will depend on how they respond to the current situation.

They are releasing themselves from the debt if they can **BALANCE** it by wanting to serve the other person and thereby end any animosity; if not, life will bring them back together in ever-closer association until it is successfully completed.

To balance these forgotten *'debts'* of the past is the only reason most individuals are brought together. People that are drawn to one other in a loving and harmonious manner have undoubtedly worked together harmoniously in the past and are therefore able to bring that much-needed quality into the world.

When someone exhibits resistance or a sense of *"being on guard"* when you meet them, it is usually because they are recalling unpleasant and discordant past associations. However, when they do, it is because of their own actions that have been set up, and the consequences can be extremely painful.

Those who locate and use the *DIVINE TOOL* that has been made available to them are fortunate. Knowing that *God's forgiveness* for the misapplication of His energy is always available to those who genuinely want it is reassuring.

The doctrine of 'eternal damnation' which was brought forth to control the people through fear, superstition and blind obedience *IS NOT TRUTH!*

Whatever the sins or past mistakes; whatever the causes of impurity and imperfection that have been set up, *THERE IS A CONSCIOUS WAY* of transmuting those errors and thus be free of them. It is the *DAILY USE of the Violet Fire of Love, Mercy, Forgiveness and Transmutation!*

Every help is offered to man when he at last understands that he is the root of all the suffering and limitations in his world and genuinely wants to *MAKE THINGS RIGHT*. Up until that time, he often acts either in rebellion against God and the situation or in submission to it, believing it to be God's Will, which is obviously untrue!

THE VIOLET TRANSMUTING FLAME

A current power source called as the Violet Transmuting Flame is capable of absorbing flawed energy and dissolving it, recharging it with Perfection. It is an act of love, mercy, and compassion that has the power to eliminate human-caused problems with the most upsetting results.

Humankind will have to confront the past causes that bring such sorrow into his life and the globe at large unless he can realise this and actively *USE this Violet Fire.*

This is what is going on in the world right now. Up until recently, the only places in the world where the knowledge of the Sacred Fire was known and taught were the Retreats of the Ascended Masters.

The year *1954* was the beginning of the **YEAR OF FREEDOM** for the Earth. It was a special time in the history of the planet when Freedom was to take its Eternal Dominion here.

It also means that the violet transmuting flame will transform the energy that surrounds humanity and the atmosphere, which has been tainted by impurity, strife, and violence. Once this is accomplished, humanity will be able to receive guidance from the **"I AM"** Presence and the Ascended Host of Light once more, granting freedom to all aspects of life.

The **Elemental Kingdom**, four-legged creatures, and all living things will eventually live as God intended His creations to live from the beginning: in love, peace, harmony, and freedom. Man will not be the only one to profit from this.

The removal of the miscreation's in your emotional, mental, etheric, and physical bodies will start when you call to your own God Presence—**"I AM"**—and ask any of the **Great Beings on the Seventh Ray** to **BLAZE** this *Violet Transmuting Flame* through you. You will feel lighter and more buoyant, your mind will be clearer, and your physical body will be charged.

As they bring this Violet Fire into action in their worlds, some pupils **SEE** it; others **FEEL** it. Regardless, once it is called forth, it does its flawless job. Despite their apparent invisibility, all the powerful abilities we employ on a regular basis are.

Using the Violet Transmuting Flame daily can also stop a lot of things from happening in your world. It should be noted, though, that if you use this flame with sincerity and something minor does happen, it does not mean that the *Violet Fire* is not working perfectly; rather, it means that your human creation is emerging more quickly than you have been destroying it.

This exercise has been described as a *"moving stairway"* that allows you to ACT by bringing the energy of the past into your present.

Using the *Violet Transmuting Flame* sufficiently to keep this energy dissipated before it can act is your task! Continue with even more resolve to dissolve **EVERYTHING** that comes to the surface for purification as soon as possible after you have used the Violet Fire with deliberate effort and feel that you are no longer disturbed by certain human characteristics and creations.

Never take the possibility of losing any momentum you have already established in this area.

Here an interlude of soft music should be inserted while the attention is directed toward the ***Violet Transmuting Flame***.

Suggested tapes for this are the *Seventh Ray and Violet Fire* Music from The Music Library of the Masters, which includes **Strauss Waltzes** *etc.*

PART 2

THE LAW OF FORGIVENESS

Although the **Violet Transmuting Flame** is essential for dissolving and transforming flawed energy, it should always be used in conjunction with a genuine sense of forgiveness for both your own and humanity's mistakes. It benefits both you and humankind when you invoke the Law of Forgiveness for all your past transgressions as well as those of **EVERY HUMANKIND.**

Never activate the Violet Transmuting Flame without first applying the Law of Forgiveness to the things that contributed to the formation of the conditions you want to purify.

When you call upon the **"I AM"** Presence of **ALL MANKIND** and ask the Violet Fire to burn through them, forgive their mistakes, and release them, it allows the **"I AM" Presence** to take action, even though it may have been centuries since it was called upon and granted permission to support that livestream. The **"I AM"** Presence of ***EVERY individual*** desires only Perfection for that individual.

The Ascended Masters perceive us differently than we see each other when they gaze upon us.

The hues surrounding us reveal what we have been feeling, and the shapes around us reveal what we have been thinking. They do not care if they perceive light or shadow.

For many of people around us, our own criticisms, resentments, depressions, and annoyances may be worse than anything else. It is necessary to transform the drab colours into the vivid ones of Perfection and the shadows into Light.

Saying **"I AM"** repeatedly throughout the day will eventually bring a lightness to your being and the world that you never imagined possible. **"I AM"** is the Cosmic Law of Forgiveness and Transmuting Flame of every mistake I have ever made, as well as the ***Cosmic Law of Forgiveness and Transmuting Flame*** of the mistakes of ALL humankind, in God's Most Holy Name.

Keep in mind that you might have previously hurt animals, birds, and other living things in addition to people. It is possible that you mistreated the intelligent beings of the Elements of ***Earth, Water, Air, and Fire***—all of which are working to become more perfect than you and I are.

We are living in the Age of Freedom! Seize the chance while it lasts! To have protection in your world during times of crisis, make a sincere attempt to correct all the faults you have ever done in your thoughts, feelings, words, and actions against every aspect of life.

From now on, make every effort to only build up causes that include perfection as one of their effects. Every bit of life that has ever been entrusted to you—which is made up of many tonnes of energy—must eventually be cleansed, balanced, and given back to God in the same condition as when it was given to you.

It is these flawed, discordant, and wicked creations—made by *MAN, NOT BY GOD*—that are acting and attempting to act everywhere that strange things are happening on Earth.

The most effective ways to stop them from acting in your reality are to call upon the Law of Forgiveness and use the Violet Transmuting Flame. When enough people engage in these activities, they can stop upsetting events from occurring all around the world.

THE LAW OF HARMONY

Everything else is based on the Fundamental Law of Life, which is harmony. Man suffers some sort of distress when it is shattered. God's pure Life Energy cannot bestow its gifts on you if your thoughts and emotions are not in constant harmony.

We are informed that the religion of the future will be the **LAW OF HARMONY,** which will be so basic that it will not require study! Humanity will be more inclined to exert self-control and deliberately place only perfection upon the priceless gift of their lives once they realise that their misery has resulted from their disobedience of this straightforward law.

Humankind wants Peace, Freedom, Love, Happiness, and Abundance, but how can it manifest for them - let alone the Earth - unless they first *GIVE Peace, Freedom, Love and Happiness* to all life everywhere?

Remember that the brain, body, emotions, and affairs of the individual generating the **HARD** feelings—hatred, prejudice, intolerance, jealously, and downright viciousness against another aspect of life—must first travel through. Simply put, war is the culmination of numerous smaller conflicts involving spouses, siblings, parents, neighbours, friends, towns, and nations!

The protection of men and nations does not require a larger army or more potent weaponry. It urges on people to seek to the God Presence **"I AM"** and the Ascended Host of Light for direction, protection, and peace, as well as to pour out enough goodwill and impersonal divine love towards one another!

Let each of us say and FEEL: **"God grant us PEACE,** and **LET IT BEGIN WITH ME!"** perfection of whatever man desires to manifest.

Your desires are formed by your mental body, which holds them there until your emotions give them energy to manifest in your environment.

By mentally storing images of the flaws they see, hear, or discuss—pictures that are fuelled by emotions and driven into manifestation—humankind has employed this process in reverse.

This energy will likewise be purified by the violet transmuting flame. Everything that has ever happened to the life stream, both good and bad, has been stored in the Etheric Body, which is the repository of memory.

When you repeatedly experience the upsetting events of the past, you allow them to reappear in your world. All these imperfect records will be transformed and dissolved by the ***Violet Transmuting Flame.***

Then there is the physical body, which has all three of the other bodies' flaws imposed and stamped upon it.

This will be altered by the Violet Transmuting Flame, which is rhythmically pulled and blazing through every organ, cell, and bodily function!

Since you are an extraordinarily complex piece of machinery and the physical body is an amazing feat of engineering, the fact that you have seven bodies should not be any more unusual than the fact that your car has many parts.

Since your car's electric system, cooling system, fuel pump, spark plugs, carburettor, and other components must all function properly for it to perform smoothly, is it necessary for all your body to be.

The Beloved Ascended Masters guide and direct us in the more effective operation of our many bodies, much as a skilled mechanic might advise you on how to improve the performance of your vehicle. Because you think and feel something every single instant, both awake and asleep, you are either constructing your Crown of Light or your karma of distress with every thought, sensation, word, and action.

How are **YOU** using **YOUR** bodies? What are **YOU** creating? The Violet Transmuting Flame is the merciful **DIVINE TOOL** which can and **WILL CHANGE EVERYTHING** in your world when it is used enough! But **IT MUST BE CALLED INTO ACTION!** It will not come forth by Itself!

Continue to apply this Activity of the Sacred Fire with vigour and enthusiasm until you and your world are free of all limitations and distress of all kinds. This will lead to your liberation.

FORGIVE ME

Forgive me, o my Presence.
Forgive me - I do pray!
Forgive all my transgressions.
Against Love's sweet way.
Oh, help me love enough.
To wipe out all mistakes of mine.
I Love You! I Love You!
Oh, help me be Divine!

Forgive them, o great Presence.
Forgive humankind we pray.
Forgive all their transgressions.
Against Love's sweet way!
Oh, help them love enough.
To wipe out all that ne'er should be.
Oh, love them! Oh, love them!
Until they are ONE with Thee!

PART 3

GROUP DECREEING

Beloved Presence of God - "I AM" in my and my own Holy Christ Self; as I invoke the Ascended Masters' Cosmic Law of Forgiveness, Forgetfulness, and the Violet Transmuting Flame of Mercy and Compassion into action in the most powerful Name - "I AM."

I command the oceans of the Violet Transmuting Fire to explore the cores and origins of the entire mass etheric records of distress that I and all of humanity have created since the beginning of time, through the misuse of God's Life and all elemental substances anywhere, at any time, and for any purpose.

By this Almighty Freeing Power and Illuminated Faith, enable and compel humanity and the Elemental Kingdom to cooperate peacefully, fulfil their Divine Plan and Vows, and swiftly transform this planet Earth into the real Holy Star of Freedom!

*This I ask in **God's Most Holy Name - "I AM"!** **Beloved Presence of God - "I AM"** in me; Ascended Master Saint Germain and all who serve in the activities of the Seventh Ray to our*

Earth; **BLAZE up,** *through and around me Your Mighty* **VIOLET TRANSMUTING FLAME,** *the Purifying Power of Di vine Love, in Its most powerful, dynamic activity.*

Transmit every one of human thoughts desires, and emotions into my being and the world, as well as any errors for which my external self bears responsibility.

Replace it with the Substance of Divine Love, Purity, and Perfection of the Ascended Master, and maintain Your supremacy in my environment and inside me forever!

In your name, and with the power of the "I AM" that is given to us, **WE DECREATE: "I AM" Angels of the Violet Fire of Freedom, Transmutation, Mercy, Forgiveness, and Love; Ascended Master Saint Germain** *and all those who serve in the Seventh Ray's activities on our planet.*

COME - COME - COME BLAZE (3) *Your Violet Transmuting Fire through my feelings! Remove all emotions of uncertainty, fear, lack and constraint, envy, impurity, discord, and hatred.*

TRANSMUTE *their causes and cores and* REPLACE *them with Your Feelings of Divine Love, Purity, Harmony, Freedom, and Perfection.*

BLAZE (3) *Your* **Violet Transmuting Fire** *through my brain structure and mental world!*

Remove and change every representation of imperfections of any type there, along with their root causes and essences. into thoughts and pictures of Beauty and Perfection.

BLAZE (3)** Your **Violet Transmuting Fire** through my Etheric Body and remove every memory of my past hurts and my imperfect, tense, and violent events, together with their root causes and essences, and **REPLACE** them with the remembrance of only **Good, Peace, Happiness, and Perfection!

***BLAZE (3)** Your **Violet Transmuting Fire** through every organ, cell function and section of my physical body, and keep it there until all signs of ageing, pain, and imperfection of any type are eliminated and transformed into my eternal youth and beauty, flawless health, boundless strength, and energy, and I am certain that my divine plan will succeed.*

I thank and bless and love You for instantaneous answer to my every Call to Light!

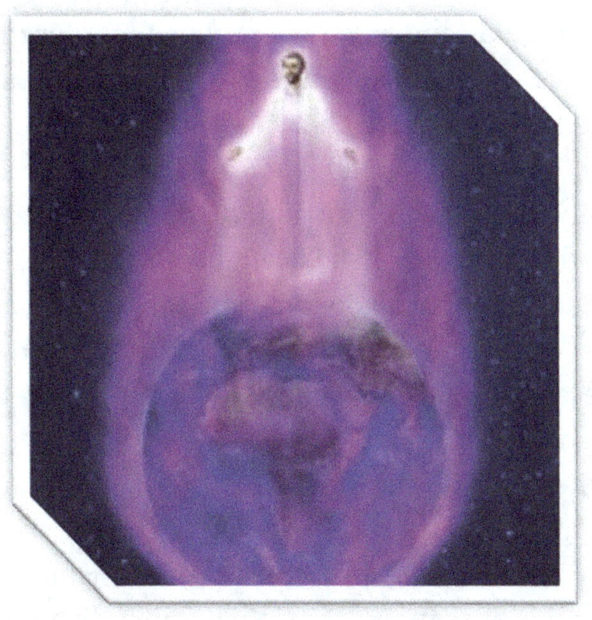

APPLICATION

In the secure environment of your own space, in the regular and rhythmic practice of Adoration to your God Self, first silence the outer self, and then shift the focus to the' 'I AM" WITHIN!

Offer it all your affection and devotion, and silently ask It to fill your body, mind, emotions, and etheric consciousness with Lighter and Love. Let your love and goodwill spread to all living things in your near vicinity as you call for its perfection. Then, call for it to spread over the entire world.

Then feel the Ascended Master Saint Germain's Presence envelop you in a Pillar of the Violet Transmuting Flame as you send Him your love and adoration. Feel this flame burn up, though, and around your physical body, eliminating any physical discomfort. It is the purest and most exquisite shade of violet. Extend this action over your city, your immediate neighbourhood, and the entire planet Earth.

Be mindful of this Blessed Violet Transmuting Flame as it surges through your mental realm, etheric body, and emotions, dissolving any "hard" emotions, tensions, or discomfort.

Feel as though God's goodness and mercy have replaced them all with kindness, love, mercy, and peace. When used sincerely and consistently throughout the day, especially three times a day in a rhythmic manner, this Violet Transmuting Flame is REAL and does produce benefits!

ACCEPT this Violet Transmuting Flame as REAL! Use it and be free!

Use music of the Seventh Ray and/or Violet Fire.

PART 4

OUTLINE FOR DIRECTOR OF CLASS

Before students arrive, the leader should light the three candles according to the Basic Manual's pattern. Before class starts, soft music should be played for at least 30 minutes. Students should remain silent and take in the atmosphere. The LEADER welcomes the pupils, then proceeds with the invocation after a brief visualisation:

We love and adore You in the Name and by the Power of Full God Reality—"I AM"—the Source of everything that exists, everywhere, and is rooted in each of our hearts and the hearts of all people! We accept that You are the One who owns and provides our life, intelligence, substance, and everything else! Enclose us in Your Love and Light, and You Might of Successful Achievement!

Prepare the path for us to constantly travel in the Path of Light by blazing Your Light and Love before us. Provide us with protection and guidance, the illumination of the truth that will free us, and guidance and direction. Let us always BE and manifest Your Divine Love, allowing it to flood through us and bless everyone we meet.

We thank You! Great Ascended Host of Light, the Messengers of God - the Ascended Masters, Cosmic Beings, Seraphim, Cherubim and Angelic Host; the Great White Brotherhood and the Elemental Kingdom; we send our Love to You! Come up in this class and help each person by doing what you see they need most to be happier, more at ease, and more obedient to the light.

We thank You!

BENEDICTION

SEALED in a Pillar of Saint Germain's Violet Transmuting Flame, Beloved Presence of God - "I AM " in us and all mankind; Great Host of Ascended Masters; Cosmic Beings, the Angelic Host and Elemental Kingdom Who have served us this day; we thank You for Your outpouring of Light and Love; we thank You for Healing, Supply, Wisdom, Protection, and Perfection, and Your Blessings of every kind.

Send them out through us for the blessing and upbringing of all life worldwide, and hold them sustained in, though, and around us. May you all experience the blessings and benediction of the Highest Living God, alongside that peace that is beyond human comprehension.

May the God of Mercy protect and guide you on your Spiritual Pathway toward Enlightenment and Freedom.

Marilena Mocanu

BLEST VIOLET FIRE

Blest Violet Fire of Freedom's Love,
Oh, blaze and blaze and blaze!
Blest sacred Fire from God above,
all raise; all raise; all raise!
Descend! Defend! Transmute and
dissolve, now free the earth by Fiery Love!
Blest Violet Fire, in Freedom's Ways,
Oh, blaze and blaze and blaze!

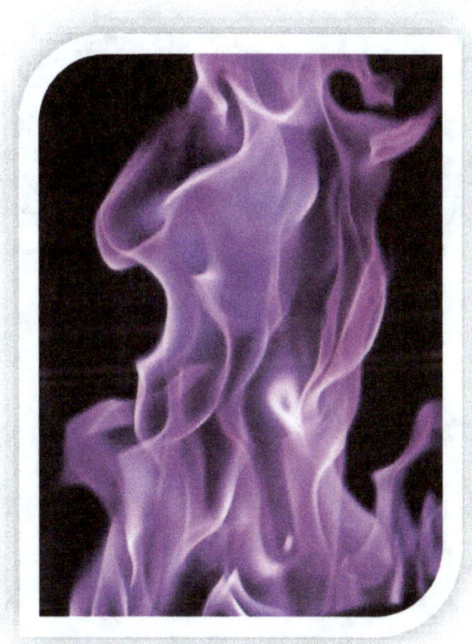

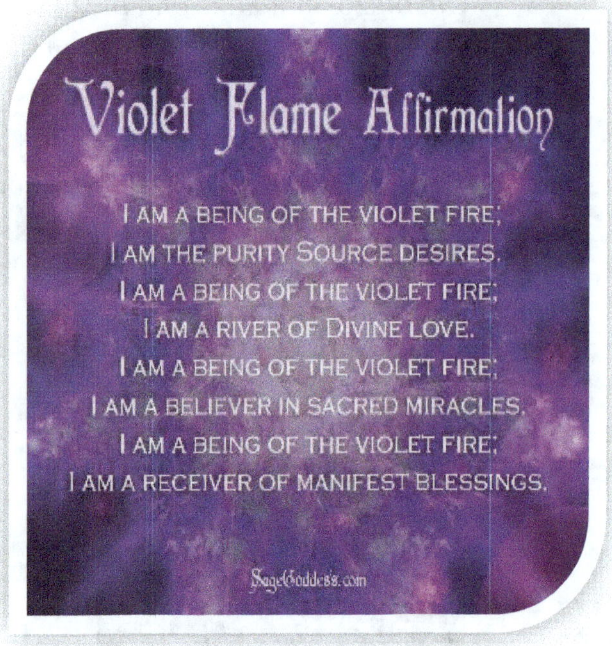

Violet Flame Affirmation

I AM A BEING OF THE VIOLET FIRE;
I AM THE PURITY SOURCE DESIRES.
I AM A BEING OF THE VIOLET FIRE;
I AM A RIVER OF DIVINE LOVE.
I AM A BEING OF THE VIOLET FIRE;
I AM A BELIEVER IN SACRED MIRACLES.
I AM A BEING OF THE VIOLET FIRE;
I AM A RECEIVER OF MANIFEST BLESSINGS.

SageGoddess.com

Affirmations

"I AM" the Life and the Resurrection!

"I AM" the Ascension in the Light!

"I AM" the Open Door that no man can close!

"I AM" *the Presence that moves acting in response to human demands, human creations, and human limitations Leave without difficulty!*

"I AM" *the Presence—the ONLY Presence that ever acts! You are the necessary condition that transforms My Perfection into discord and human limitations!*

"I AM" *ever pouring forth into your mind and body, the fulness of My Light and Perfection! You are continuously requalifying My Perfect Energy into something you do not desire out of your own free choice and qualifications!*

Test Me! *turn your face to Me—your God—and let the Light from Every discordant item that you have drawn about yourself throughout the ages is* *forever removed from your mind, body, home, and world as my face shines upon you!*

"I AM" the Consuming Flame that, when called into action, dissolves, and consumes forever your miscreation's!

Considering *these remarks, everyone should realise for the last time that they are not obligated to keep their mistakes because they have already been made. "I AM" the Presence that sets you FREE!*

*"I AM" the Presence that must have your call to liberate and set **FREE My Mighty Energy**, to Purify and Perfect your world. May these words serve as a living fire in your mind that you will never forget, clearing your mind of all obstacles and bringing order to your environment!*

"I AM" the Presence that speaks!

"I AM" the presence that gives you the impression that the money you need is a gift and a substance from me—in the form of money—and when I give, the Freedom of Divine Love acts.
Then know that I AM the ONLY GIVER of all money that has come to you or will come to you in the

*future! Therefore, when you call to Me, I respond to you in ways you would not imagine. When you call, you cannot be denied money for necessities the **"Mighty I AM Presence"** into action, for **I AM** the **ONLY INTELLIGENCE** that can act!*

*"**I AM**" the ONLY POWER that can act!*

*"**I AM**" the Enfolding Light of Divine Love—forever active — that releases your needs via eternally sustained Divine Love!*

*"**I AM**"! (3) BY GOD I KNOW "I AM" THAT*

*"**I AM**"! AND THE GOD AUTHORITY EVERYWHERE I MOVE! "Mighty I AM Presence"! Annihilate all human authority from this Earth! for "I AM" the Divine Authority of the Sacred Fire! "I AM" BY GOD I KNOW "I AM" THAT "I AM"! the Cosmic Being of the Seven Mighty Elohim and the Unfed Flame, which CONDUCTS the annihilation of all human power! "I AM" the Authority of the Sacred Fire that COMMANDS the Divine Plan fulfilled here by the Cosmic Love, Protection, and Perfection that blesses all!*

*"I AM"! (3) BY ALL GOD'S LOVE I KNOW
"I AM"! the Invincible, Irresistible Magnetic
Pull upon the energy of my outer self by the
Great Central Sun Magnet; the Pull upon me
attention, and upon my energy, into the
Realm of Perfection, which is my Higher
Mental Body's World of Invincible Power,
Substance, and Activity of the Sacred Fire.
the Invincible Authority of my "Beloved
Mighty I AM Presence"!
 "ALMIGHTY I AM"! (3)*

Use for one week:

*"MY WORLD IS THE INVINCIBLE VICTORY OF
THE GREAT CENTRAL SUN MAGNET'S LOVE!*

*"BELOVED MIGHTY I AM PRESENCE"!
CHARGE the Invincible Victorious Love of
the Great Central Sun Magnet into me
world's physical activity! into everything
and everyone I encounter—the physical
world, everything, the atmosphere,
the Powers of Nature!
I DEMAND the Invincible Love from the
Great Central Sun Magnet BLAZE surround
me and serve as this week's attitude!"
"ALMIGHTY I AM"! (3)*

Use daily:
"I GIVE CONSCIOUS RECOGNITION AND ACCEPTANCE, *that the Great Central Sun Magnet's Love, and the Ascended Masters' Feeling of the Violet Consuming Flame from the Violet Planet, is the Magnetic Power drawn in and around me, to consciously concentrate a Focus around my physical form! It becomes a reservoir, a powerhouse, a sun presence of the concentrated Love and Feeling from the Violet Planet in and around me, and it does for me what only that Love can accomplish when I pour its Presence into my affairs!*

"I AM" *filled and surrounded by the Violet.*
Consuming Flame, which is giving me the
feeling that Great Central Sun Magnet's
Love that draws me up into the Purity of the
Violet Consuming Flame: likewise,
wherever I go, I become an Outpost of Its
Action! **"ALMIGHTY I AM"!** *(3)*

"BELOVED MIGHTY I AM PRESENCE" AND GREAT HOST OF ASCENDED MASTERS! *CHARGE the Violet Flame Love of the Great Central Sun Magnet's Power into me Electronic Circle, which develops into a Force Reservoir that draws only Perfection to me! Bring me the Great*

Central Sun Magnet's Magnificent Power of Violet Flame Love, which will instantly repel everything else? and draw all that is of God to me! **"ALMIGHTY I AM"! (3)**

"I pour my Love to my **"Beloved Mighty I AM Presence"** *and the Great Central Sun Magnet, and ask Its Love Enter and embrace me as the Healing Love of the Universe! CHARGE everything that vibrates around me, to become the Purifying Flame, which releases the substance of the outer self from the discord and impurity imposed upon it!"* **"ALMIGHTY I AM"! (3)**

"I SEND MY LOVE TO THE VIOLET FLAME! *and I call Its Power forth from the Great Central Sun Magnet To control my universe, my being, and my electronic circle!*
I move ahead in the Great Central Sun Magnet's Power of Violet Flame Love—
Master over all!
"ALMIGHTY I AM"! (3)

"I AM" THE LAW *of the Great Central Sun Magnet's Health of that Love of Immortal Purity! I CHARGE this external self with those magnetic currents that attract*

*external action that results in permanent
Health in me and all under this Radiation!*
"ALMIGHTY I AM"! (3)

"I AM" THE LAW of Immortal Victory
*overall, in this world, by the Great Central
Sun Magnet's Immortal Love, which pulls
everything in creation towards me to help
me triumph! I send Its Living Presence and
Flame in the physical octave, and I demand
Its Perfection manifest here forever!*
"ALMIGHTY I AM"! (3)

"I AM" THE LAW *of the Eternal Illumination of
the Victorious Christ, and the Great Central Sun
Magnet's Love draws It to me from the Heights of
Creation! "I AM" the Visible, Tangible Illumination
of this which I desire! Right now, and forever!*
"ALMIGHTY I AM"! (3

" *I* **live, move,** *and possess my presence in a
Blazing Sphere of the Violet Consuming Flame's
Presence! and the Angels of the Violet Flame
about me, make it a permanent part of my
everyday activities for all time!*
"ALMIGHTY I AM"! (3)

Abundance

"I AM" here and *"I AM"* there! **Money floods** to me from everywhere, as a glad free Gift of Love, tax Free for all Eternity; everything will be used under the guidance of Ascended Master Wisdom in the Service of the Light. at all times, to produce and expand only Perfection, eternally sustained!
"ALMIGHTY I AM"! (3)

"BELOVED MIGHTY I AM PRESENCE" AND GREAT HOST OF ASCENDED MASTERS! You seize control of my economic circumstances and maintain Ascended Master God Control, Supply, and release of all the money I desire, now and forever!
"ALMIGHTY I AM"! (3)

"BELOVED MIGHTY I AM PRESENCE"!
Do not ever let me be short of money again!
Observe how the awareness of want.
is eradicated out of the whole Universe, so
no part of Life can ever again think of lack
not lack for any good thing; but rather make
productive use of everything, and hold
Ascended Master Invincible Perfection,
eternally sustained and ever expanding!
"ALMIGHTY I AM"! (3)

"BELOVED MIGHTY I AM PRESENCE"!
*Come forth now in Thy Full Ascended
Master Power, and release to the Children
of Light Thy Full Supply of every good thing,
including Riches and Money! Note that
there is nothing positive that someone
under this radiation lacks! Open Your
Treasure House and supply all with an
abundance of money, food, clothing,
buildings, equipment, and everything they
desire; and keep it Invincible and Free from
everything erroneous, eternally sustained
and ever expanding!*
"ALMIGHTY I AM"! (3)

**"BELOVED MIGHTY I AM PRESENCE," ALL
GREAT BEINGS AND POWERS OF LIGHT!**
*Sweep everywhere in our channels of finance!
Annihilate any recommendations or requirements
that may cause us members to experience
economic difficulties or fear or injustice of any
kind! Charge all money and collateral in us Land
with Beloved Saint Germain's Power of the Violet
Consuming Flame and the Unfed Flame in their
Threefold Activity; and everywhere that money or
collateral goes,* **COMPEL! (3)** *it to produce*
Perfect
Balance, Freedom, and Divine Justice *to*

everyone inside our boundaries, as well as the infinite Supply of all good things to us people everywhere; and through it compel Divine Justice forever!
"ALMIGHTY I AM"! (3)

"BELOVED MIGHTY I AM PRESENCE" AND GREAT HOST OF ASCENDED MASTERS!
Release into my hands and use today!
$_________ as a Glad Free Gift of Love!
Give me Ten times the amount as I want, and see that I use it all in the Service of the Light forever!
Remove all obstruction, its cause, effect, record and memory in my emotions, which could cause a delay or prevent this Instantaneous Release into my use! I thank Thee Thou dost always answer my Call instantly!
"ALMIGHTY I AM"! (3)

"BELOVED MIGHTY I AM PRESENCE" AND ALL GREAT BEINGS AND POWERS OF LIGHT!
Blaze! blaze! blaze! *"The Light of God That Never Fails," into every aspect of our people's financial lives, with such Overwhelming Power and Ascended Master Pressure of Light that It **ANNIHILATES!** (3)*

*Every time money is used destructively
within our Land! Replace it by the Ascended
Masters' Divine Justice, Purity, Balance,
and Blazing Perfection to everyone who
seeks the constructive way of Life—
Invincible and Free from all wrong forever!*
"ALMIGHTY I AM"! (3)

**BELOVED JUPITER, FORTUNA, AND LORD
MAHA CHOHAN! (3)**
*Through and to us Thy overwhelming, Ever-
expanding Supply of everything positive,
including money now in our hands, forever
expand!*
**Expand! Expand! Expand!
Descend! Descend! Descend!**

**THE UNFED FLAME OF A THOUSAND SUNS IN
THE POWER OF THE "THREE TIMES THREE"!
(3)**
*All of us are exposed to this radiation
worldwide, and it reaches our hands and is
released. Your Limitless, Overwhelming,
and Ever-expanding Supply of every good
thing, including money, and see we use it
only as You would, and make it instantly
and forever expand!*
Expand! Expand! Expand!

Descend! Descend! Descend!

ARCHANGEL MICHAEL AND LEGIONS OF LIGHT! (3)
Thy Limitless Money to us forever expand!
Expand! Expand! Expand!
Descend! Descend! Descend!

POSSESSION, SUPPLY, AND MONEY OF A THOUSAND SUNS! (3)
Through and to us forever compel! (3)
By the Power and Light of a Thousand Suns! (3)
For in the Ascended Masters' Eternal Supply, we do forever dwell! (3)
"ALMIGHTY I AM"! (3)
"I AM"! "I AM"! "I AM"! BY ALL GOD'S LOVE I KNOW "I AM"!
The Visible, tangible presence of everything I need for external use! "I AM" the Ascended Masters' Consciousness of God's Limitless Supply of every good thing, and my infinite usage of that Supply everywhere I move, Invincible and Free from all wrong everywhere forever! "
"ALMIGHTY I AM"! (3)

"IN THE NAME, AUTHORITY, AND THE SACRED POWER OF THE GREAT COMMAND! I DEMAND whatever is necessary in me outer use, be allowed to create and maintain my unbreakable freedom and eternal independence of, and forever untouched by the money beast, all its claws, and the so-called power, powers, and limitations of the physical world! **I demand** *this by the Great Cosmic Unfed Flame of Love Supreme, in Obedience to the Ascended Masters and Their Cosmic*
Victory forever! **"ALMIGHTY I AM"!** *(3)*

"I AM" the Resurrection and the Life of the overwhelming, boundless, invincible Supply of all my blessings from the first two Golden Ages, and it again comes forth to serve me and fulfil the Ascended Masters' Divine Plan Their Way! Right Now! this instant and forever!
"ALMIGHTY I AM"! *(3)*

"I AM" the full acceptance of the Limitless Money and everything good have been brought into Saint Germain's possession and used Foundation, the Staff, and all who serve the Light; for the Expansion of all Beloved Saint Germain's "I AM" Activities throughout the world! Right Now! this instant and forever, and

I DEMAND THIS MANIFEST NOW! (3)

FLOOD US WITH MONEY! (3)
"Almighty I AM"!
God, take Command!
Right now, today!
In Your Perfect Way!
All our bills now pay!
In Victory to stay!
All Perfection hold sway!
God Almighty, hold sway!
Beloved Saint Germain's Freedom
now forever hold sway!
I DEMAND THIS MANIFEST NOW! (3)

FLOOD US WITH WEALTH! (3)
"Almighty I AM"!
From God's own Hand!
Throughout our Land!
God, take Command!
In God we stand!
We insist and demand!
By our God Command!
Right now, today!
In Your Perfect Way!
On God's Love Ray!
All our bills now pay!
In Victory to stay!

All Perfection hold sway!
God Almighty, hold sway!
Beloved Saint Germain's Freedom
now forever hold sway!
I DEMAND THIS MANIFEST NOW! (3)

RELEASE BILLIONS AND BILLIONS AND BILLIONS OF DOLLARS!
Billions, "Almighty I AM"!
Billions, from God's own Hand!
Billions, cash in our hands and use today!
Billions, At this moment, God's Way!
Billions, Your success over and for us will always reign supreme!
Billions, Your Freedom through and to us forever hold sway!
Billions, Your Protection through and to us forever hold sway!
Billions, Your limitless Supply through and to us forever hold sway!
I DEMAND THIS MANIFEST NOW! (3)

THROUGH THE "BELOVED INVINCIBLE FIERY VICTORIOUS MIGHTY I AM PRESENCE" WHICH "I AM," AND THE COSMIC CHRIST'S INVINCIBLE FIERY VICTORIOUS HAND AS OF A THOUSAND SUNS FROM MY "BELOVED MIGHTY I AM PRESENCE," THAT OF ALL

MANKIND, ALL THE ASCENDED MASTERS, THE COSMIC BEINGS, THIS SYSTEM OF WORLDS, THE GREAT ANGELIC HOST, AND EVERYONE WHO DIRECTS THE SACRED FIRE!
I DEMAND, I COMMAND, I INSIST, AND
"I AM" THAT "I AM PRESENCE" WHICH COMPELS, COMPELS, COMPELS, AND
FOREVER MAINTAINS, that "I AM" the Cosmic, Electrifying, Expanding Power that makes our money grow, and grow, and grow, and become the Limitless Supply for which we call!
"ALMIGHTY I AM"! (3)

"BELOVED MIGHTY I AM PRESENCE," GREAT HOST OF ASCENDED MASTERS, GREAT COSMIC BEINGS, GREAT ANGELIC HOST, AND ALL WHO GOVERN SUPPLY TO THE EARTH!
**EXPAND OUR MONEY! (3)*
"ALMIGHTY I AM"! (3)
I DEMAND THIS MANIFEST NOW! (3)

**Also use:*
BLESS OUR MONEY!
PROTECT OUR MONEY!
PROTECT OUR WEALTH!
PROTECT OUR SUPPLY!

"I AM" all the Wealth, Money, Opulence, and Supply of every good thing required for the Expansion of all Beloved Saint Germain's **"I AM"** Activities, made visible immediately, both now and forever.; Eternally sustained, ever expanding, Protected, and All-powerfully active, and
I DEMAND THIS MANIFEST NOW! (3)
 KEEP *OUR MONEY ROLLING IN! (3)
"Almighty I AM"! (3)

From God's own Hand! (3)
By the billions, every day! (3)
Tax free to stay! (3)
From God's Precipitating Ray! (3)
Controlled, protected, sustained, and
expanded to forever hold sway! (3)
For the Ascended Masters' Divine Plan
fulfilled, the Ascended Masters' Way to
forever hold sway! (3)
I DEMAND THIS MANIFEST NOW! (3)
**Also use:*
GOD'S SUPPLY
GOD'S WEALTH

RELEASE INSTANTANEOUS PRECIPITATION THROUGH US! (3)
"Almighty I AM"! (3)
By God's own Hand! (3)

By God's Great Command! (3)
And all Thy Miracles each hour! (3)
By all Mighty Victory's Power! (3)
By all Mighty Cyclopia's Power! (3)
By all the Lord Maha Chohan's Power! (3)
And double It through us all each hour! (3)
I DEMAND THIS MANIFEST NOW! (3)

THROUGH THE "BELOVED INVINCIBLE MIGHTY I AM PRESENCE" WHICH "I AM"!
I CALL TO THE GREAT HOST OF ASCENDED MASTERS, THE COSMIC BEINGS AND GREAT ANGELIC HOST; THE "MIGHTY I AM PRESENCE" AND HIGHER MENTAL BODIES OF ALL HUMANKIND; ALL GREAT BEINGS, POWERS, AND LEGIONS OF LIGHT! COME! COME! COME! IN YOUR VISIBLE, TANGIBLE, ASCENDED MASTER BODIES! RAISE YOUR COSMIC SWORDS OF BLUE
FLAME OF A THOUSAND SUNS FROM THE GREAT CENTRAL SUN THAT TRANSCENDS EVERY HUMAN CONCEPT! and
CHARGE! (3)
BLESS! (3)
PROTECT! (3)
SUPPLY! (3)
PERFECT! (3)
DIRECT! (3)

AMPLIFY! (3)

MULTIPLY! (3)

EXPAND! (3) *all Beloved Saint Germain's*
"I AM" Activities— His Homes, Offices, Supplies, Property, Equipment, Business Activities, and all that He has created for the Light's Expansion, to the glory of His servants!

Bless, protect, supply, and charge the Staff; the Messengers; all our invincible, God Victorious attorneys and accountants: All of us, including ourselves, are exposed to this limitless radiation. Invincible Abundance of every good thing— including money, homes, buildings, equipment, transportation, communication, and everything required for the worldwide.

Expansion and upkeep of Beloved Saint Germain's "I AM" Activities! Put everything in our hands and put it to use immediately! Keep it Eternally sustained, ever expanding, world engulfing, and All Powerfully Active always—on time, ahead of time, at the right time, all the time! I thank Thee it is done, and **I DEMAND THIS MANIFEST NOW! (3)**

"I AM" God's Invincible Presence!

"I AM" God's Invincible Power!

"I AM" God's Invincible Hand of Flame!

Supplying all each hour!

"I AM" God's Invincible Presence!

"I AM" God's Victorious Power!
"I AM" God's Invincible Hand of Flame!
Stopping all lack this very hour!
"I AM" God's Invincible Presence!
"I AM" God's Victorious Power!
"I AM" God's Invincible Hand of Flame!
Precipitating God's Invincible Wealth,
each instant of each hour!
I DEMAND THIS MANIFEST NOW! (3)

SUSTAIN! (3) and expand the Ascended Masters'
Every good thing is infinitely available to everyone
below this radiation, in, though, and around them,
a billion times more each instant of each hour!
and KEEP ALL THE BILLS, DEBTS, AND
OBLIGATIONS OF ALL UNDER THIS
RADIATION PAID IN ADVANCE TODAY AND
FOREVER! (3)
"ALMIGHTY I AM"! (3)
Hold the picture of the word PAID on everybody's
bills.

SWEEP THE COSMIC LOVE OF THE ALL-
SUPPLYING CHRIST! (3)
In, though, all around and to everyone
beneath this Radiation, a billion times more

*each instant of each day, with lightning speed each instant of each hour! and **KEEP! ALL THE BILLS, DEBTS, AND OBLIGATIONS OF EVERYTHING UNDER THIS RADIATION, PAID IN ADVANCE TODAY AND FOREVER! (3)***
"ALMIGHTY I AM"! (3)

***RELEASE THY SUPPLY! (3)** a billion times more each instant of each day; maintained and protected indefinitely, in, though, and around, and to all under this Radiation, with lightning speed each instant of each hour!*
"ALMIGHTY I AM"! (3)

***EXPAND OUR SUPPLY! (3)** of all the positive things in, around, and to everyone beneath this radiation, a billion times more each instant of each day, with lightning speed each instant of each hour!*
"ALMIGHTY I AM"! (3)

*I **DEMAND** the **Invincible Eternal Purity! (3)** that **Never, Never, Never fails! (3)** to **KEEP! (3)** all exposed to this radiation **Invincibly Supplied! (3)** with all*
God's Invincible Money! (3) with all God's Invincible Wealth! (3) with all God's Invincible

Supply of everything positive! (3) with all God's Invincible Opulence! (3)
with all God's Invincible, Limitless Legions of **Ascended Master Friends, Protectors, and Defenders of all under this Radiation, everywhere forever! (3)**

I DEMAND the Invincible, **Eternal Purity! (3) Never! Never! Never fail! (3)** *to* **KEEP! (3)** *all the bills, debts, and obligations of all under this Radiation Invincibly* **PAID! (3)** *in advance* **today and forever! (3)** *and* **never! Never! Never fail! (3)** *to* **KEEP! (3)** *all under this Radiation invincibly out of debt everywhere forever! (3)*
"ALMIGHTY I AM"! (3)

I DEMAND AND "I AM"! (3) our Invincible God Supply of God's Invincible Money direct from God, and the full settlement of all obligations, debts, and obligations for everyone protected by this Radiation, Paid in advance today and forever! by the Mightiest Violet Flame Love in the Universe!
"ALMIGHTY I AM"! (3)

GOD, THE "BELOVED MIGHTY I AM PRESENCE," BLAZE! (3) *Your Fiery Hand and Miracle Love of the Universe into the money supply as well as all other people under this*

radiation; and keep ten times more money in our hands and use at all times than we will ever require; and fulfil Your Divine Plan, Your Way, through and to us all forever!
"ALMIGHTY I AM"! (3)

GOD, blast us free! *God, keep us free, for all eternity, from any financial lack!*
God, blast us free! God, keep us free from all lack of any good thing for all Eternity!
"ALMIGHTY I AM"! (3)

"BELOVED MIGHTY I AM PRESENCE" AND GREAT HOST OF ASCENDED MASTERS! UNLOCK THY TREASURE HOUSE! (3) *to everyone under this radiation indefinitely; and keep and use 10 times more of anything useful that we may ever require or desire—including Riches and Money as a Glad Free Gift of Love, tax free for all Eternity in every nation of the world; fulfilling the Ascended Masters' Divine Plan the Ascended Masters' Way, in all we ever do or contact until all are Ascended and Free!*
"ALMIGHTY I AM"! (3)

I DEMAND *Everything in our worlds and beings must be the victory of the Sacred Fire of the Ascended Masters' Eternal Purity and Boundless*

Supply of every good thing from the channels—the right channels—You know can come to us now, and Invincible against all evil forever!
"ALMIGHTY I AM"! (3)

"BELOVED MIGHTY I AM PRESENCE" AND ALL THE ASCENDED HOST! BLAZE Your Cosmic, Fiery Christ, Miracle Love of the Universe into our Money Supply as well as everyone else under this radiation! Keep ten times more in our hands and use than we will ever require; and fulfil Your Divine Plan Your Way through and to us all forever.
"ALMIGHTY I AM"! (3)
"I AM"! (3) I know "I AM" FREE! (3), free from all money lack forever!
"ALMIGHTY I AM"! (3)

I DEMAND all this Money for which I call!
I DEMAND all this Money that now pays all!
I DEMAND all this Money that blasts
all Free!
I DEMAND all this Money that makes all
*see, the Hand of my **"Beloved Mighty I AM Presence"** responding to me, compelling God's Immortal Victory of the Ascended Masters' Divine Plan fulfilled, Their Way, in everything we do or meet.*

in the physical world until everyone is free
and ascended!
"ALMIGHTY I AM"! (3)

"I AM" THE RESURRECTION AND THE LIFE of
the Ascended Masters' The first divine method of
bringing about God's provision of all good things,
a billion times more each instant of each day, with
lightning speed each instant of each hour!
"ALMIGHTY I AM"! (3)
COME! (3) billions of Legions of Ascended Master
Friends of the Sacred Fire in the Great Central
Sun—in rapid descent into Earth's physical
structure! And complete the payment of all the
bills, debts, and obligations of all under this
Radiation, a billion times faster each instant of
each day! *"ALMIGHTY I AM"! (3)*

*"BELOVED MIGHTY I AM PRESENCE"! IN THE
NAME OF THE ASCENDED JESUS CHRIST! I
DEMAND* the Ascended Jesus Christ Immortal
Supply now made manifest!
"ALMIGHTY I AM"! (3)

I DEMAND AND "I AM" all this money for which I
call, visible and tangible in our hands and use
today!
"ALMIGHTY I AM"! (3)

I DEMAND AND "I AM" the All-Christ Fire Authority of all the Boundless Supply for which I call!
"ALMIGHTY I AM"! (3)

I DEMAND AND "I AM" ALL THE COSMIC WEALTH OF THE VIOLET CONSUMING FLAME FOR WHICH WE CALL! (3)
"ALMIGHTY I AM"! (3)

"I AM" here! "I AM" there! God's "I AM" Money flows into us from everywhere, fulfilling the Ascended Masters' Divine Plan, the Ascended Masters' Way, in all we ever do or contact until all are Ascended and Free! *"ALMIGHTY I AM"! (3)*

"BELOVED MIGHTY I AM PRESENCE," ALL GREAT BEINGS, POWERS OF SACRED FIRE, THE COSMIC LIGHT, AND THE MIRACLE LOVE OF ETERNITY! BLAZE! (3) the Fiery Hand of Your Miracle Love into all our financial activities; and *MANIFEST! (3)* in our hands and use, right now, ten times more money than we will ever require; and keep all the bills, debts, and obligations of all under this Radiation, paid in advance today and forever!
"ALMIGHTY I AM"! (3)

"BELOVED MIGHTY I AM PRESENCE" AND ALL THE ASCENDED HOST! *Take out of me and keep out of me; take out of all under this Radiation and keep out of all under this Radiation all of which could impede or postpone our bringing forth the Invincible Perfection and Supply of everything for which we have called and hold it Invincible against all evil forever!*
"ALMIGHTY I AM"! *(3)*

"I AM" the Ascended Masters' Law of Forgiveness and Consuming Flame of all inharmonious action and human consciousness, that Never, Never, Never fails! To Sweep the Cosmic Concentration of the Cosmic Purification, Under this radiation, everywhere, through everything! And COMPEL the annihilation of all problems, lack, and limitation, all delay and human creation, that Never, Never, Never fails! To KEEP all the bills, debts, and obligations of all under this Radiation, paid in advance today and forever, everywhere throughout Creation! **"ALMIGHTY I AM"!** *(3)*

IT IS ALSO THE REQUEST OF JESUS AND SAINT GERMAIN, THAT THOSE, WHOSE INNER SIGHT IS OPEN AND WHO SEE WHAT TAKES PLACE DURING A GROUP MEETING,

REFRAIN FROM TELLING OTHERS WHAT THEY SEE; AS EACH INDIVIDUAL IS EXPECTED TO KEEP HIS PERSONAL EXPERIENCES GUARDED WITHIN HIS OWN HEART AS A SACRED, SILENT, SECRET GIFT TO HIM. IF THIS IS NOT DONE, THE BLESSING TO HIM IS LOST, FOR WHEN HE TELLS HIS EXPERIENCES TO OTHERS, HE RELEASES THEIR ENERGY INTO THE SURROUNDING ATMOSPHERE AND HENCE, HE DOES NOT RECEIVE THE HELP INTENDED FOR HIM.

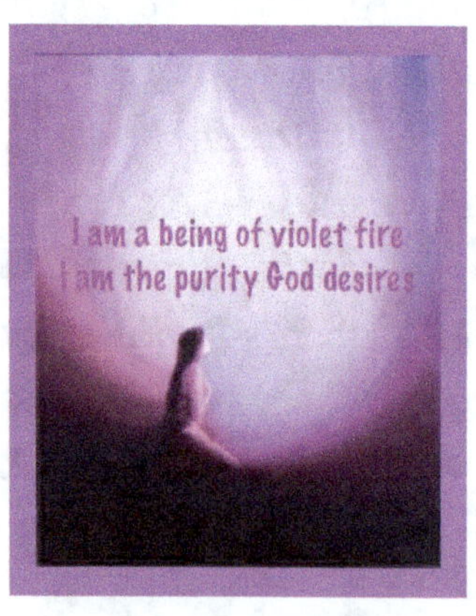

About the Author

Marilena Mocanu is an author, spiritual guide, and advocate for personal transformation. Helping people realise their full potential and embrace a life of prosperity, meaning, and inner peace is her life's work. Marilena has devoted her life to studying the wisdom of the Ascended Masters, especially Saint Germain, whose teachings have had a considerable influence on her life. She has an ardent desire for spiritual development and empowerment.

Her books, *The Path to Prosperity*, *The Magic Words "I AM"* and *Daily Meditations with the Ascended Masters*, are all part of her journey to share the transformative teachings of **Saint Germain**.

In **The Path to Prosperity**, Inspired by Saint Germain's teachings, Marilena investigates the concepts of prosperity and self-determination. This book provides a spiritual road map for attaining success in all spheres of life, including spiritual, emotional, and financial. To assist readers overcome challenges and realise their aspirations, Saint Germain's insights on the Violet Flame and its capacity to transform negativity into positive energy are crucial.

In *I Am the Magic Words,* Marilena explores the transformative potential of spoken words and affirmations. In keeping with Saint Germain's teachings on the value of mental alchemy and the application of affirmations to effect good change, this book explores how our words have the power to influence our reality. Through mindful language and a mental shift, the book gives readers the ability to shape their own world.

Daily Meditations with the Ascended Masters combines what Marilena has learnt from previous Ascended Masters and Saint Germain. The purpose of this compilation of meditations is to assist readers in everyday communication with the divine teachings and energies of the Ascended Masters. Readers are encouraged to experience spiritual liberation, healing, and harmony with their highest purpose by implementing these daily activities.

The teachings of Saint Germain serve as a profound inspiration for all Marilena's publications. She feels that his teachings on empowerment, transmutation, and spiritual liberation are essential for anybody looking to grow and change. Through her writing, Marilena provides readers with resources to assist them live out these lessons, overcome obstacles, and enter a life of happiness, prosperity, and spiritual enlightenment.

Marilena's desire to share the great wisdom of Saint Germain and her own self-discovery are reflected in her work. People can connect with the divine wisdom that has guided her life through her works, which provide a path to spiritual awakening. Marilena thinks that anyone may discover their way to success and undergo long-lasting change by adopting the principles of Saint Germain.

Associated Books

May you be interested??

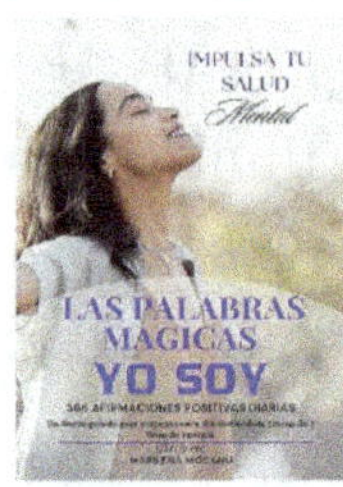

ASIN : B0CPBV6Q6W

Publisher : Independently published

Language : Spanish

Paperback : 123 pages

ISBN-13 : 979-8868270703

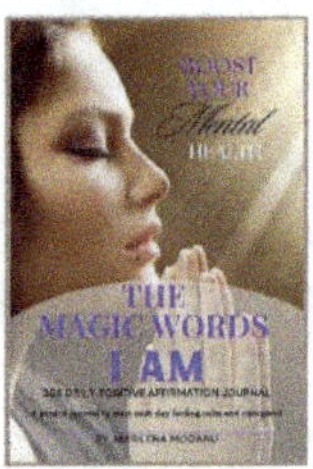

ASIN : B0CNWJMQ25

Publisher : Independently published

Language : English

Paperback : 123 pages

ISBN-13 : 979-8867418472

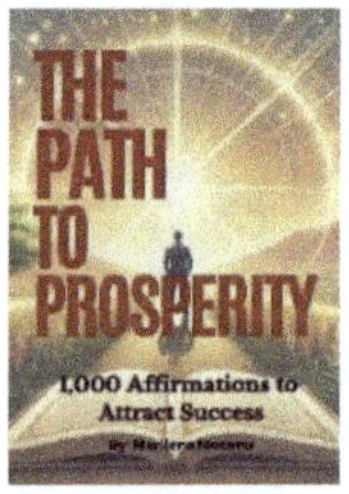

ASIN : B0DJDBBF5Y

Publisher : Independently published

Language : English

Paperback : 249 pages

ISBN-13 : 979-8340871091

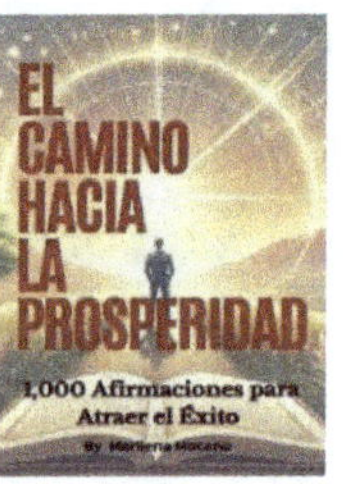

ASIN : B0DKXVGRCH

Publisher : Independently published

Language : Spanish

Paperback : 265 pages

ISBN-13 : 979-8342491433